UNFOLDING THE TENT

Advocating for Your One-Of-A Kind Child

ANNE ADDISON

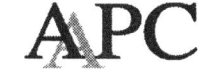

Autism Asperger Publishing Co.
P.O. Box 23173
Shawnee Mission, Kansas 66283-0173
www.asperger.net

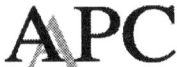

© 2005 by Autism Asperger Publishing Co.
P.O. Box 23173
Shawnee Mission, Kansas 66283-0173
www.asperger.net

Publisher's Cataloging-in-Publication
(Provided by Quality Books, Inc.)

Addison, Anne.
    Unfolding the tent : advocating for your
one-of-a-kind child / Anne Addison.
    p. cm.
    Includes bibliographical references and index.
    LCCN 2005929652
    ISBN 1-931282-80-3

    1. Children with disabilities—Education—United
States. 2. Attention-deficit-disordered children.
3. Autistic children. 4. Child rearing. 5. Success in
children.   I. Title.

LC4031.A33 2005   371.9
                          QBI05-600103

This book is designed in Adobe Garamond and Akzidenz Grotesk.

Printed in the United States of America.

Dedicated to the teachers and staff of
North Street School and Eaglebrook School

At birth our divine potential is folded up in us
like a tent. It is life's purpose
to unfold that tent.

— *Abess Hildegard von Bingen (1098-1179)*

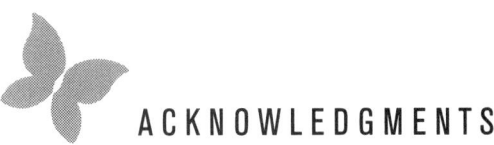

ACKNOWLEDGMENTS

The ideas, concepts and philosophies in this book have largely been shaped by the incredible teachers, coaches, friends and stray angels that have wandered into the path (and hung in for the journey) of our family. There is no better living definition of a high-functioning team than those that I have partnered with at North Street School, Eaglebrook School, Cooperative Education Services, Trinity Church and the BASH team, and Kanakuk Kamp. I have been kept on the path of middle school years by Andy Kilroy, who goes beyond any and every expectation of a remarkable teacher. I am heartened always through the wisdom and love of the First Presbyterian Church and its Tuesday Bible Study, Trinity Church and First Fridays and the Wednesday Prayer Group, who have taught me that God is everywhere, even at the kitchen table. Sue Moreno is a fastidious editor who brought this book into focus, and Kirsten McBride a thought-provoking editor that always challenged me (in a good way). Lauren Graessle once again brought my book to life through her design skills. Sally Eberhardt is probably the world's best psychotherapist. There are no better people to be on a team with than Bill Horn, Charles Smith, and Dan French. I am blessed daily by my friendships with Valerie Craig, Lynn Hagerbrant, Sheri Pasqualoni, and Carlene Safdie. My husband, John, and children, Sarah and Jack, keep me from taking myself too seriously and remind me what life is all about.

CONTENTS

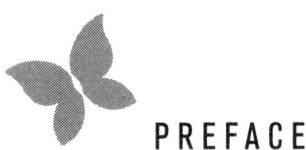

PREFACE

About the time that our one-of-a-kind child[1] was school age, some nagging questions began to settle in the back of my mind: "Where is Jack going to end up?" "What will we need to do to make sure that he gets to the best place that he can be?" "And what kind of path should we encourage him on?" From where we had already been, I knew that I couldn't just let nature take its course.

I did a little more thinking. Correction. I did a lot more thinking! And I went to conferences, interviewed top professionals, and surveyed parents. I wanted to know what made the biggest difference in the life of a child who has special needs in terms of "making it" – whether the "it" was college, a job, pursuing a talent, or developing friendships.

Whenever I spoke about my family's experience and parents saw how much Jack[2] has overcome difficulties, parents would ask me what we did that achieved such dramatic change. They didn't want just situation-specific fixes. They wanted a blueprint for helping their own children reach their potential.

The roadmap that I had created to move Jack forward I had borrowed from the classic strategic planning process used in business: define a vision, set goals, develop strategies and tactics, and off you go. For a child-oriented strategic plan, the plan had to encompass all the aspects of his life and reflect who he was, right at his core. It had to honor his individuality but be mindful of his limitations. The result is what I call the Life Map, and I am excited about sharing it in this book.

– A. A.

---

[1] The examples and context of this book are directed towards children with neurological, learning, behavioral, attention and developmental disorders. This is the population I am referencing when I say "special needs."

[2] Jack is like a Chinese menu, having a feature of this and a feature of that. As he has gotten older, it mostly resembles ADHD with features of Asperger Syndrome. Jack is eleven years old and just started middle school this past year.

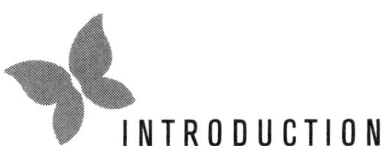

INTRODUCTION

For typical children, moving through the cognitive, emotional, and physical developmental stages of life is a natural progression. With the right people and experiences put in their path, for the most part, they continue to move along. But for most children with special needs, if we want them to become responsible, capable, and happy adults, we need to chart a path from where they are today to where we – and they – hope they will end up.

Determining who you want to become and what you want to do in life requires knowing yourself, what you like and don't like, what you can and can't do. It also requires a certain amount of social smarts. Because, like it or not, the road of life is paved with relationships and interactions. How absolutely unfortunate then, that some children have trouble in both of these areas – introspecting and relating to others. They don't think much about their inside selves at any given moment, never mind thinking ahead a month, a year, or a lifetime. And they pretty much live in a state of social confusion. Their hearts are in the right place, but their social senses are not.

If your child is going to make it in life, there is a greater chance that he[3] will succeed if there is a roadmap to guide him; one that draws on his strengths and minimizes his challenges. You will have to be intentional about his future. You will need to teach him to be intentional as well, being mindful of what he needs to be successful and being able to access the tools to get there.

The Life Map presented in this book will help you define a vision and goals for your child's future and provide the tools to achieve them. Depending upon your child's cognitive and emotional abilities, you will need to figure out how much

---

[3] For ease of reading, references to your child will be made using the pronoun "he"; if you have a daughter, just substitute "she" when you read "he."

he can participate in this process. As he matures, his role should increase until he is eventually able to take the lead in creating his own Life Map.

The Life Map is a framework for helping a child reach his potential and become the best he can be. If it's a clerk at the local grocery store, let's help him become the one with the biggest smile and the largest helping hand. If it's a herpetologist, let's figure out how to teach him effective listening skills so that he can be part of a research team.

Supporting your child with the skills that he needs does not mean that you are defining his dreams for him. If your child is high functioning, he will have his own dreams. Your role is to look at what competencies he needs to achieve them and help him get there.

Competencies go beyond technical skills. In fact, technical skills may be the least of your worries. If your child is succeeding in school, he will probably be able to get through the necessary technical training and education to reach his goals. You have to think about the social, relational, emotional, and practical skills he will need – defining what they are and creating opportunities to practice, practice, practice them so that they become competencies. If his school performance is less than successful, then your work will include this component as well.

And that's where this book comes in. Part I presents the Life Mapping model. This overview will help you to understand the concept of the Life Map and how it comes together to help your child reach his highest potential. In order to implement the Life Map, it is important to fully understand your child. Part II will help you to see your child from his perspective. But in addition to understanding your child, there is you. You are a critical influence in your child's world. The attitude and mind-set with which you approach your role in helping your child reach his highest point is everything. Part III focuses on this self-searching. Since there are usually many others, in addition to you, who support your child and who are part of your child's team, Part IV concentrates on effective team building and skills to make sure everyone pulls in the same direction. Finally, Part V shows you how to implement the Life Map.

Throughout the book you will encounter exercises. You may be tempted to skip them, but please don't. They are there to encourage the kind of thinking that is necessary for you to develop a well-thought out Life Map for your child.

Now your work begins. You are probably the engine that got your child over his first set of hurdles. You probably understand him better than anyone. So who better to dig in and help him over the next set? You have more experience, more practice, more vested interest, and more love for him than anyone else. It's not easy, but parenting, and especially parenting a child with special needs, never is. There will be setbacks and disappointments along the way. That's just part of the process of life.

Following is an excerpt from a letter that we received from Jack's teacher and advisor several weeks after Jack began middle school.

"Jack really is beginning to show his personality, and as we have a great abhorrence of cookie-cutter kids, we like the fact that he is so independent and outspoken. For instance, in class today I was explaining that academic competitiveness at the school is not really encouraged. That we judge each student by his or her individual progress, not by how they measure up to other students.

Having said that, I handed out the vocabulary workbooks, where each student works at his own level. Of course, they started comparing their levels immediately. I went through the explanation again. Jack raised his hand and said, 'I don't go for all that mind-control stuff. Of course, it is better to be in a higher book.' Inside I was chuckling (thinking, there's my little rationalist), but I tried to assure him that I don't play 'mind-control' games and am as honest as I can be, given the circumstances."

You've got to love a kid like that. Carving a path, being conscientious and careful to match your child's temperament and personality to the environment and culture, whether it is school, an activity, or the structure of your home, pays off. You'll see it the minute your child's tent starts unfolding.

PART I

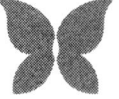

WHAT IS LIFE MAPPING?

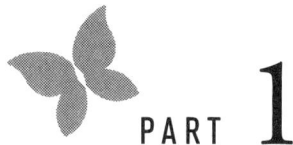

PART 1

WHAT IS LIFE MAPPING?

Life Mapping is a process used to realize a person's fullest potential by drawing on his strengths and interests and working on his challenges. Companies go through processes like this all the time. They identify their competitive edge, take a look at what barriers are in the market, and come up with goals and a way of reaching them that will satisfy both consumers and stockholders.

Maybe you've done Life Mapping (although you probably haven't called it that) for yourself – getting to know who you are and what you're good at, setting goals that relate to that, and then establishing a way to accomplish them. I'm not suggesting that you won't have a perfectly satisfactory and fulfilling life if you don't do Life Mapping. But for children with neurological, learning, behavioral, attention, and developmental challenges, being intentional and thoughtful about who they are and what they need throughout their lives will improve the odds that they will live satisfying lives.

Pretend that it is your friend's birthday and you have offered to throw her a party. You ask her who she would like you to invite and what she would like for dessert. Tossing Dr. Atkins to the wind, she says breathlessly, "Triple chocolate mousse cake with extra filling – and don't skimp on the frosting." Determining what you need to do to put the party together, from invitations to cake, is the *plan*.

Having your friend enjoy a wonderful party and that delicious cake is your ultimate goal, vision, dream, and desire. To make the cake, you look in your kitchen cabinets and see that you've got a couple of eggs and some vanilla. That's the starting point. You go to the grocery store and buy the rest of the ingredients, and then proceed to make the cake. From finding out what ingredients were on hand to spreading the last of the butter cream frosting on the cake is *process*. In fact, all of the actions that you take between coming up with the party idea to holding the event are part of the process. The actual party is the endpoint, the goal.

The *people* are everyone involved in the event, from the birthday girl to the clerks at the stores where you shop to the guests and yours truly. They are the ones that carry out the process.

The birthday party could be thought of as a mapping experience: making a *plan*, using a *process* that leads you toward the goal, and working with *people* in the process. These three things are at the heart of Life Mapping.

THE THREE ELEMENTS OF LIFE MAPPING

Let's take a closer look at the elements behind Life Mapping: the players, the process, and the plan.

1. THE PLAYERS

The child, the parents, and those who regularly work with your child make up the foundation of the Life Mapping model. At the center is the child. That seems obvious. You might even say to yourself, "Of course, it is all about him. I spend half of my waking minutes thinking, worrying, making calls, setting plans, and fussing about him." It is a full-time job, no doubt. But doing the work requires understanding the child. Life Mapping will only be as strong as the foundation is. And the foundation starts with the child. Understanding your child means more than knowing what the doctors and other professionals have told you that he "has." It means knowing many different aspects of him. By nature of his challenges, it is often hard to get close to or understand your exceptional child. But you need to keep trying, because the more you understand your child, the better you'll be able to help develop a Life Map for him.

The next part of the foundation is the parent(s.) You're the one(s) who provide the overall support for your child. You might think this support focuses on how your child functions at home, but since you are his coach, mentor, and case manager, your influence extends into every part of his life. You have a huge impact on the success of your child's Life Map, so it's vital to understand yourself. The more you know yourself and are aware of how your behavior and attitudes impact your child, the more effective you can be.

The folks who support your child on various teams (school, medical, etc.) make up the final piece of the foundation. We have all been on teams that are effective and teams that are not. Effective teams can move mountains, let alone move toward goals. The dysfunctional team cannot. The better the team functions, the more your child will benefit. We will look more closely at the nature of the players and their roles in Part II.

2. THE PROCESS

In Life Mapping, there are many factors that influence, impact, and drive the process. But for our children, the two primary factors are the parent(s) and the team that supports the child. These individuals work closely and on a regular basis with the child. Their interactions with the child may be positive, negative, or neutral, but they all have a huge impact. Part III will address process in its various dimensions.

3. THE PLAN

Defining goals and having a plan to reach those goals provides a structure for helping you stay focused and mindful that what you are working on are the things that you should be working on. And in the case of helping a child reach his potential, you have to know what specifics that, when added together, constitute that potential. If you want your child to reach his highest potential, you need to define what that might look like and then develop the steps that are needed to achieve it.

A BIRD'S EYE VIEW OF LIFE MAPPING

LIFE MAPPING AT WORK IN REAL LIFE

It is Sunday morning, and I am way more stressed than I should be. I am, or rather my family is, in a race with time. This is a race that they normally lose, which annoys me to no end, since I am the driver. I've called the children at least twenty times to come down to breakfast, but each has a reason for why they can't join me. Sarah is busy doing and redoing her hair. This I understand. I was once thirteen and remember spending hours following as closely as I could the directions in Teen *magazine to get the hairstyle they promised could be done in five easy steps. Jack is another story.*

Jack is a child who doesn't just march to the beat of his own drum; he leads his own parade. All this individualization is not totally his fault. Jack has special needs that challenge time management, organization, and focusing skills, just to name a few. There are electrical disconnects and minute discrepancies in his brain chemicals that make getting himself dressed, fed and ready for church by 10 a.m. a major challenge.

With new resolve, I turn up my voice a notch to show my two children that I am not kidding. I grab the two plates of French toast and yell up the stairs that they will now be having breakfast to go – which really irritates me. That means that the car I diligently had washed yesterday will now have a sickening sweet smell by 11:30 a.m., thanks to two eggy, sugary pieces of toast baking in the backseat for several hours. Not a good start to the day.

When we finally get to church I lean down to Jack and for the second time today try to keep my annoyance to myself, but I hear it creeping in as I tell him, "I want you to sit with us today, Jack. And I mean it."

The church is fairly full, a sign that the Christmas season is coming, so I head straight up the stairs to the balcony where the overflow crowd and those who aren't sure they really want to be here this early in the morning sit. Sure enough, Jack waits until I have stepped onto the balcony, then turns and heads back down again. I motion to Sarah to take a seat in the first row so that I can get a good view of the sanctuary and track Jack. Just as the entrance hymn ends and the congregation begins settling in, I spot Jack, methodically walking up each aisle looking for his very good friend and fellow herpetologist, Ned. It is the same thing every week.

Jack's self-imposed nickname is Eskimo Man, and he looks like one, hunkered down in his bright yellow down coat with its mammoth hood covering most of his head. I watch Jack make his way around the church as the rest of the congregation follows the request of the minister to bow their heads and pray. When I raise my head, Jack has disappeared from sight.

He is missing during the baptisms of two babies and the standard prayers, and he doesn't head up to the altar with the other children when the children's sermon is announced. The Lord alone knows where Jack has gone off to.

As we were leaving church, a friend of mine came up to me. "Jack was so helpful at the door today. He insisted on holding it for everyone and helping the older people find their seats."

I looked at my friend. "Great, but wouldn't it have been nice if he would have come in and sat with me just once?" I asked.

"Oh, but how sweet it is of him to help out," she reminded me.

True, very true. So do I give him a consequence for not obeying me or let it slide? On the one hand, it was very nice that he helped the ushers with the door. For a child who sometimes has trouble thinking about the other guy, assisting the church members was a big deal. On the other hand, he deliberately disobeyed me. Didn't give my words a second of thought.

Driving home, I thought about some of the goals that we were working on with Jack. "Following directions" was one of them. That has been on the list since day one. But so has "connecting with people," which is why I had let Jack start sitting with his friend at church months earlier. Not to mention that it was a good incentive to get him to church.

I know my child. Once Jack gets into a pattern, he has difficulty breaking it. And there really wasn't anything wrong with him sitting with his friend, except that he sometimes gets too chatty. The real reason that I wanted Jack to sit with us was that I was getting tired of having the family spread throughout the church. I wanted it to be more of a family event. I had been asking him for several weeks, but sitting with Ned was now a pattern that he had to continue.

If I wanted to, I knew that I could explain to Ned's parents that I wanted Jack to sit with our family and that they would help me make this happen. Jack looks up to Ned's father and would listen to him if he told Jack it would be best if he sat with us. But I thought it would be more empowering in the long run if I could get Jack, and perhaps Ned, invested in finding a solution. Jack was old enough to understand my desire to have the family sit together even if it wasn't what he wanted to do. He could see there were solutions that would satisfy my need and his as well. For example, Ned could sit with our family one week and Jack could sit with his family the next. That would both satisfy my need and Jack's desires, and at the same time he would be working on an important social skill. But to get to this new format meant that I had to broaden my concept of family church and stop being "stuck" in how I was looking at the situation.

Sometimes, an issue comes along that cannot be compromised. But if you look at it objectively and rationally, you may find that what seems like a "have to" is more about your need to have things your way than it is about getting your child to the "right way." There are often more roads than the one that you planned for your child or the family to travel on.

This is basically how Life Mapping works. Keeping your eye on the goals, understanding your child, having supportive people around, and being adaptable along the way. With this overview in mind, let's go to where it all begins – with the people, and specifically, your child.

THE BOTTOM LINE

- Life Mapping is a process-oriented approach to life that focuses on developing skills and competencies.

- The child is at the center of the Life Map. Understanding the child is the first step to creating a Life Map that works for him. Don't limit his future by looking at where he is today. Rather, think in terms of your child's potential.

- The way that you and your child's team "see" your child will significantly impact how he sees himself and what he believes he can (or can't) do.

PART II

THE PLAYERS

Understanding Your Child and Yourself

SECTION 1

UNDERSTANDING THE CHILD

CHAPTER 1

DIAGNOSIS, SYMPTOMS, AND LABELS

Sometimes Things Are as Clear as Mud

My friend Laurie, a highly capable and life-filled woman, had a second pregnancy that was quite uneventful – just the way you like them. At her "time," Laurie and her husband drove the five minutes to the hospital where her labor continued. Laurie was huffing and puffing, thinking about nothing but the end of this hard labor and focusing on the finish line, when suddenly she felt the air in the delivery room change. People were rushing around, and soon she felt herself being wheeled into a different room and prepared for a Cesarean section. Something was going wrong, but everything got blurred before she could ask what. In a rush came her second child, Samantha, and in that same rush Samantha was whisked off to another room along with Laurie's husband. A few minutes later, Laurie's husband returned, alone.

"Laurie, you know how we always say we are so blessed to have such a good, good child in Michael? And how we were worried how the next child would handle having such a jewel of a big brother? God has given us a child who will never have to compete with Michael …" That is how Laurie learned she was the mother of a child with Down's Syndrome.

THE DIAGNOSIS IS JUST ONE PIECE OF THE PIE

A diagnosis is just one piece of the battery of information you use to try to come up with the best plan for your child. A good diagnosis begins with qualified professionals doing the testing and other evaluations, which, for many disorders, is part art and part science.

Brain chemistry is a fluid, living thing and, therefore, is constantly changing, unlike a disease that has fixed biological roots. What this means is that we have to be on our parental toes, observant of new behaviors and emotions that may be indicators of a new disorder[4] revealing itself or an old one worsening.

Even when you think you have figured out what it is that your child has, you can't necessarily find a book that describes him to a "tee" – which would help guide you in developing a treatment plan. This is because the total constellation of each child is unique although many of these disorders share some similarities. What Asperger Syndrome, autism, or attention deficit hyperactivity disorder (ADHD), for example, looks like in one child is often remarkably different in another.

If you are reading this book, you probably have a child who has already gone through some battery of tests and has received one or more diagnoses. Stay on your toes, though, because what you see at age two is not necessarily what you'll see at age ten, twenty, or fifty. Some of the issues you see in your child's younger years will be overcome, but the core disorder, if it has been properly diagnosed, typically remains.

Being a watchdog is no easy feat. For starters, you're not always sure whether what you are seeing is the emergence of a new problem, a reaction to something in the child's environment, or just a bad day. And if you, one who is familiar with the rhythm of your child, have trouble telling, how can people who see your child infrequently tell what is real and what is a reaction?

I desperately wanted to go to the annual CHADD (Children and Adults with Attention-Deficit/Hyperactivity Disorder) conference this past year. But since John, my husband, had a business trip and would be away at the same time, it looked

---

[4]   The term "disorder" in this book refers to learning, neurological, behavioral, attention, and developmental disorders.

doubtful. Truth be told, he would need an extra pair of hands to help him even if he were home. That's just the way it is.

We don't have any regular babysitters now that our children are older, but I did manage to beg a lovely, very capable, thirty-something woman to stay with our children for two nights. I arrived in Miami and quickly unpacked, hoping to make the most of my forty-eight-hour getaway. Armed with lined paper and pen, I headed out for a quiet dinner before the conference the next morning. Bringing my cell phone was the evening's downfall. The salad course had not even arrived when I got my first phone call from Mary Beth, the sitter.

"Anne?" I heard a quavering voice on the other end. "The kids are fighting over who gets to sleep with the cat. I think you're going to have to hospitalize me," she laughed nervously. Of course, there is truth in every jest. I had Mary Beth walk me through the evening up to that point; it was now bedtime, which is never the easiest time in our house. When we finished debriefing, we concluded that it had been a pretty good evening after all.

In truth, the evening had gone much better than similar events in Jack's earlier years. Fighting over who gets to sleep with the cat only happens a couple of times a year in our house. In fact, not much sibling fighting goes on at all. So, did Jack have an anxiety issue with someone other than his parents sleeping at his house, was it just one of "those days," or did his sister provoke him and he had nothing to do with initiating the battle? This is not easy stuff to sort out.

If someone like Mary Beth, who has logged a lot of time working with children and knows my children well, can spend a few hours and get a certain impression of Jack, what slice of your child does the psychologist or psychiatrist get when he or she spends a couple of hours and completes an assessment? How much is your child's personality and temperament affected by the stranger, the new setting, and the unfamiliar activity? For each child, the answer will vary.

The inability to make an air-tight diagnosis does not mean that you should dismiss getting your child evaluated. Well-respected, conscientious evaluators use a number of diagnostic tools that can give valid information that leads to an accurate diagnosis and gives you important insights into your child's strengths and weaknesses.

It is extremely useful to the diagnostician if you can provide her with input from people who interact with your child on a regular basis, both individually and in a group setting. If the evaluator doesn't suggest it, you should suggest he gain such supplemental information. When deciding whom to get input from, don't just choose people your child knows well; select them based on what role they play in his life. This will help the evaluator to assess your child more accurately.

How Often Should My Child Be Evaluated?

The Individuals with Disabilities Education Act (IDEA) requires that any child with an individualized education program (IEP) be reevaluated every three years.[5] In general, this seems to be a good timeframe. However, if your child has shown a significant change in behaviors, temperament, or anything else that is causing you worry, do not wait for the three-year mark or any other predetermined time.

How you go about investigating concerns depends upon the nature of what seems to be happening. Based upon what you (and others) are observing, ask the question, "What information do we need to make a better treatment or program decision?" Once you have identified what information you need, you can determine who is in the best position to obtain or provide that information. The school team and others who work regularly with your child will have observations that can provide you with good information to help you make these sorts of decisions.

---

[5] IDEA is a federal law. reauthorized in 2004 with roots in Public Law 94-142, that became a federal law in 1978. You can find the full IDEA at www.ed.gov/policy/speced/guid/idea/idea2004/html.

How Important Is a Diagnosis? Can't We Just Treat the Symptoms?

Testing done to arrive at a diagnosis is largely based upon symptoms. A proper diagnosis is important because it gives you a general assortment of symptoms that can then be examined more carefully. One way to look at your child is to go underneath the diagnosis and analyze which of the symptoms included in the diagnostic criteria are most pronounced. Simple test scores may not provide the most important information for guiding your plan. Understanding the symptoms underlying the diagnosis is critical.

In my first book, *One Small Starfish* (2003),[6] I presented a simple way for parents to get a handle on which symptoms are most significant for their child by having them rate the presence and level of behaviors in their child every half hour for a period of time. This is an excellent method for parents and professionals working with the child to objectively see what symptoms are most present during the day, to identify patterns, and to assess the severity of individual symptoms in relation to each other. It moves you from looking at the child as a diagnosis to seeing him in terms of his specific symptoms.

Be Open to New Concerns at Each Stage, However Painful It May Be

In the fall of Jack's fifth-grade year, his last year in elementary school, my husband and I decided that the very large middle school in our district would not be the best next step for Jack, so I set out to investigate private schools within a four-hour radius. The first school interview was nothing short of a disaster. From Jack's bored demeanor in the admissions waiting room to his casual attitude in the classrooms he visited (the least of which began with his introduction of himself as "Joe from Hawaii"), his behavior was questionable.

Upon reflection, I realized that Jack's day-to-day social skills had become solid because he was operating in a world where each situation had been scripted and almost every incident was predictable. We had to train for broader, basic social skills that would provide him with guidelines for how to act in new situations. Then it would be up to him in each new situation to draw on his repertoire.

---

[6] *One Small Starfish* (Arlington, TX: Future Horizons, 2003).

Ignoring whatever issues that crop up and cloud the child's ability to function in the world is not an option if you want your child to stretch beyond the challenges he was born with. Regardless of what they are – academic, behavioral, attentional – they somehow will touch every aspect of a child's world. Identifying your child's central issues and acknowledging a diagnosis, even if the child only reflects certain elements of it, is part of the preliminary work that must be done before you can begin developing his Life Map. You cannot generate a plan if you don't know what you should be focusing upon.

DON'T HIDE THE DIAGNOSIS

Not wanting to label a child has often been the reason why parents hesitate to get their child tested or keep testing results to themselves rather than sharing them with the school, teachers, coaches, and others who work regularly with their child. This is a mistake.

When I began the search for a middle school for Jack, I first identified schools that I had heard would accept children with mild attentional or behavioral needs. Before contacting the schools and asking more about their requirements, I networked my way to parents of students attending each school. In this process I was given Mrs. Ross's name and telephone number by a local support group coordinator. When I met with her, Mrs. Ross told me that her son had Asperger Syndrome and that he had been accepted at St. Mark's.

"I thought they only take children with learning disabilities and mild ADHD at St. Mark's," I remarked, curious to learn how she had convinced them that her son could manage the work.

"Oh, I didn't *tell them anything* about Stevie!" Mrs. Ross laughed. "They would never even have looked at him if I had said he came with a label."

This didn't seem right to me, but maybe I was naive, with one school rejection already to our credit. "So, how is Stevie liking school?" I proceeded.

"Well, things aren't going as well as I'd like. The other children are mean to Stevie. I feel like I'm in the assistant headmaster's office every week with one issue or another," Mrs. Ross responded, clearly annoyed.

So who was fooled? The school or Mrs. Ross – not to mention Stevie? If a child has a diagnosis that you feel is correct, it does no one any good to hide that information.[7] If a school will not consider a child because of his disorder, that means that it doesn't have the accommodations or interest to help him, even if he is admitted. Putting your child in a situation where he will not have the support he needs doesn't do him, or you, any good.

A diagnosis and a careful look at symptoms provide important information that helps you understand your child's needs in order to determine the best treatment plan and school program for him. Being able to look honestly at the issues and challenges your child faces is a critical part of truly understanding him.

LABEL THE CHILD AND HE WILL LIVE UP TO THAT LABEL

It is easy to attach a label to a child. As children, we all knew who the teacher's pet was and who caused her grief. Each of us, to some degree or another, had a label.

To see a parent openly talk about his child's disorder right in front of the child, as if he were invisible or immune to the conversation, is disheartening. Talking about the child as a label can subtly stick a child with victim thinking. That is, the child begins to see himself as his label.

There is a big difference between keeping teachers, coaches, and others who regularly interact with the child aware of his issues and repeatedly telling the child, verbally and nonverbally, "You are your label." Imagine someone telling you that you had poor eye-hand coordination. How would you feel about your gym class? You'd be ready to sit on the bench before the class even began.

STAY ON TOP OF MEDICATIONS (IF IT IS PART OF THE TREATMENT PLAN)[8]

If medication to control attention or behavioral symptoms is part of your child's treatment program, it must be constantly watched. Sometimes it takes a fair amount of trial, error, and careful adjustment to get the medications right. Some

---

[7]   In the spring of 2003, the Family Educational Rights Privacy Law (FERPA) was passed, designed to protect the privacy of individuals. As a result of this legislation, as the parent you need to give written authorization to the school and professionals you work with to allow them to speak to another professional about your child.

[8]   This does not presume that every child needs medication. Whether or not medication can be helpful in addressing your child's symptoms is something that your child's doctor and you should thoughtfully discuss, after proper testing and diagnosis.

have to reach a specific level in the bloodstream to become effective and must be maintained at that level to continue to be effective. Others, such as certain stimulant medications, are measured by the immediate impact that is observed in the child's behavior. Whatever medication protocol your child's doctor recommends, be sure to observe carefully that the medications are addressing the symptoms they were designed for.

Measuring the efficacy of medications should be part of the routine for your child. Puberty, weight gains, and the ordinary changes in brain chemistry due to maturation will impact how medications work, requiring regular adjustments. The doctor who administers the medications should be assessing them every six to nine months, depending on how stable things are at each point in time. However, an office observation gives only the narrowest slice of your child's day-to-day emotional health, social progress, and school performance. Consider asking those who work daily with your child and who are part of your team to provide their impressions so that the doctor can get the fullest picture possible. For example, a teacher's input on the child's classroom behavior would be an important component. An easy-to-use tracking tool is provided in my book *One Small Starfish*.[9]

As your child matures, he should be part of the medication evaluation as well – as long as you are confident that he is giving you honest feedback. You can begin this self-awareness by pointing out behaviors to him that are being effectively treated by his medication. If he has a day when he has forgotten it or can't take it, take the opportunity to point out any behavioral differences (from the days when he is on the medication). This is the beginning of teaching him to develop his own self-awareness and understanding of the effect his medication has on his body and his actions.

BEGIN AT THE BEGINNING

Be tenacious and turn over every stone until you are comfortable that your child has the correct diagnosis and, more important, that the issues and deficits that are tripping him up are clearly understood. As he grows, both from an organic perspective and as a result of his experiences in the world, your child's symptoms

---

[9] (Arlington, TX: Future Horizons Publishing, 2003), pp. 338-340.

will change. By keeping people who work with him focused on his needs and concerns instead of resting on a diagnosis, you ensure that the appropriate issues are being worked upon.

The better you understand who the child is, the better you can help him. But that is just the beginning. If you want the most effective plan possible for your child, you will need to dig deeper and try and see the world as he does. In the next chapter we will take a look at how we might do that.

THE BOTTOM LINE

- Looking at your child from both a diagnostic and a symptomatic perspective is the only way to get a complete picture of who he is. Few children fit neatly into a pat diagnostic description. Looking at both diagnosis and underlying symptoms will give you the fullest grasp of who your child is from a medical perspective.

- Try not to think of your child in terms of labels. With media from newspapers to movies using individuals or fictional characters to show what a person with a typical diagnosis looks like, a narrow image of your child is conjured up for others and perhaps, unknowingly, for you and your child.

- Medications must continually be monitored to determine their effectiveness for the child. Since the kinds of medication we are discussing are intended to relieve symptoms that interfere with your child's behavior, observing him in his environment is a good way to see how well the medication is working.

CHAPTER 2

Seeing the World as Your Child Sees It

You Say Black, I Say White

My husband and I had a heated discussion last night. He disagreed with our mayor's recent push to ban smoking from bars in town but felt it made sense to enforce not smoking in restaurants. I was mad and disappointed that my husband, who usually lines up with me on issues of individual liberty, didn't have the same opinion as I did. But in a split second of divine wisdom or inspiration, I decided to let the discussion go. It wasn't important that I win my husband over to how I saw things in the world of smokers versus nonsmokers.

Did you ever wonder how some people are so good at seeing another point of view and figuring out compromises even when two positions are very different? This seems to be a natural gift for some, but for others, it takes active training in the art of communication and negotiation. By the time we are adults, many of us expect, or at least want, our spouses, and those whom we are close to, to be able to discuss tricky situations reasonably. But children, and that's all children at one stage or another, come at life from a "me first" perspective. The way they learn to eventually see others' perspectives is through experience and training. Who of us hasn't taught our children the age-old adage of The Golden Rule, for example?

Unfortunately, seeing things from another person's perspective is one of the toughest things for children with social challenges. But just because they aren't born with the ability to learn and assimilate such social lessons doesn't mean we can forego trying to teach and train them. Understanding and accepting someone else's point of view is fundamental to building relationships; if you expect your child to develop meaningful relationships, you must teach this skill to him and train him how to use it.

To succeed, you must approach the child from his starting point until he is able to "hear" what you have to teach him. This doesn't mean that you have to accept his me-first positions until then. But you do have to understand how he processes and interprets information.

How We See the World

We "see" the world in three ways: emotionally, physically, and verbally. We take in and process information from our emotional center, and that impacts our response. In the smoking-in-public-restaurants incident earlier, the tone of my husband's response and the content of what he said cast an emotional color on the discussion. The physical way in which we see the world isn't just looking at what is in front of us. It is also how we read someone's body language and non-verbal language. Finally, we see the world by what people say to us, through the words they use and how they use them.

All young children are unable to read social cues. However, a typical child will usually listen to your explanation and respond to you, imitating your lead or doing what you suggest. Conversely, most children with developmental, attentional, or behavioral disorders are likely not to notice or to ignore you. Talking louder or faster, giving out punishments, or threatening, does not help them "see" things differently.

To effectively communicative with them, you need to adjust to *their* way of seeing. Once you see how they see, you can approach them from an angle they are comfortable with, with a long-term goal of working to reshape how they view the world.

Know Your Child's Starting Point

Jack and I used to get embroiled in heated discussions (okay, flat-out arguments) every day. I thought he just liked to be disagreeable. It started from almost the day he was born. I said, "Time for your nap," and he said, "I'm not sleepy." I said, "You need to share," and he said, "I'm happy playing by myself." I thought he was operating out of a selfish, "life is about what feels good to me" point of view. And in a way, that's what he was doing.

It wasn't until I understood that Jack's way of seeing precluded him from flipping a dial to look at things from any other perspective besides his own that I realized it wasn't that Jack *wouldn't* see things my way; it was that he *couldn't*. He simply didn't have the intuition or inclination to consider someone else's point of view. He was perfectly content in his own world.

This realization profoundly influenced the way I subsequently saw Jack and worked with him. When you realize that someone isn't taking three of the four muffins off the plate to be greedy and selfish but that he is only thinking about what feels good to him, you can be frustrated, but you're unlikely to be angry at the person.

With typical children we often provide a simple explanation based on a simple principle, such as "Take just one muffin so Sally and Charlie can have one, too. It is important to share with our friends and treat them like we want to be treated." Most children want to be liked and understand The Golden Rule at a young age. Unfortunately, the child with compromised social reasoning often can't get past what he wants to do right now. He doesn't think about how the children who wouldn't get a muffin might feel.

If you have been methodical in the diagnostic process and relentless in picking apart what is going on with your child, you are in a good place to now sort out how he sees the world. Things might have been fuzzy in the preschool and early elementary years, but by late elementary school and beyond, when children's cognitive abilities are engaged, you will have a clear idea of how your child sees the world.

We went into New York City recently to meet one of my friends from out of town and her two children, who are identical in age and gender to our two children. Jack knew that this was an important day to me. I adore this friend and hadn't seen her in four years. She is a mother extraordinaire, from her daily bread baking to her involvement in her children's school and extracurricular activities.

We chose to meet for lunch in a rather fancy restaurant; I knew it would be a bit of a challenge for Jack, but my friend and I wanted the children to see "classic New York City." Jack and I had made a risky decision to hold off on his medication so that he would have an appetite (one of the side effects of his medication is loss of appetite so Jack typically does not eat lunch). It was a dangerous decision, but I weighed the alternative of Jack being bored and not hungry and decided to take the chance. Jack managed to murmur "hello," but from there he became The Bread King.

A basket of very crunchy, very hard-to-eat rolls was in the middle of the table with a dish of butter next to it. Had I been more alert, I would have asked the waiter to remove the basket right away, as I knew from past experience what could happen. What could happen, did. Jack spent the next thirty minutes of getting-to-know-you conversation in bread surgery. The first roll, he cut off the top, scooped out the center, and stuffed the middle with butter, then stuffed as much as he could into his mouth. Both my friend and I made a few attempts to suggest that Jack "break off a piece and butter that" (as I have said at least a million times before to him), but Jack seemed deaf. The next roll he approached with a "dice 'em" strategy, cutting the bread into very small pieces with the help of two knives. Maybe he was trying to show us that he had heard us earlier suggest smaller pieces. From there, he consumed two pieces of flat bread, heavily lathered in butter.

My friend was wonderful. She was very nonchalant and accepting of Jack's behavior, but she consistently leaned over to make suggestions that would bring him back in line. She did so respectfully and matter-of-factly, with a bit of humor and grace and absolutely no sarcasm or negativity.

Later, I asked Jack why he had used such poor manners with the bread. Had he felt pressured, did he forget his manners, or was he just trying to annoy me? He had *no clue* what I was talking about. Although we had been gently trying to correct his behavior throughout the incident, he was so absorbed in his own world that our suggestions had not registered with him. What had really happened was a number of things – the place was too big and too noisy and he was too nervous about meeting and making a good impression on my friend – so as a result, he defaulted to behavior that was comforting to him.

I would not have handled this situation so well a few years earlier. I would have been frustrated and perhaps had to leave the table. In fact, I did that two years earlier.

When Jack was in third grade, I decided it was time for a mother-son winter vacation. Jack had been pleading all winter that I take him ice fishing, since fishing is one of his passions that normally had to rest during the winter. Except for the fact that the ice-fishing hole turned out to be a gangster hangout, our weekend in Quebec City was going well. After six hours of fishing in a fake lake with only a converted trailer/bar for warmth and standing in the cold with frozen corn on the end of our rods, and no fish in sight, we were ready for a good dinner. Jack likes a variety of foods so I felt that the restaurant I had picked would be a winner.

Down we went in the outdoor "elevator" to the windy, charming, seventeenth-century streets of Quebec. We ducked into a little restaurant where a table for two was waiting. I have figured out that if you get to a restaurant early, not only can you get a table but you don't have to bite your nails worrying about what your child might do that could disturb those trying to have a real dining experience. So there we were at 5 p.m. We made it past Jack's latest fetish — covering the top of a candleholder so that the candle is robbed of oxygen and extinguishes — and had moved to Jack ordering one of his favorites — a dish of mussels. I should have known we were going to have one of "those" evenings when Jack approached his meal by systematically opening the mussel shells, removing the meat, and piling it on a separate plate for later consumption. Not only did this look messy, it was messy.

I don't remember what we were discussing but the subject of hats came up. The next thing I knew, Jack was down on the carpet with his linen napkin in tow. Over and over again, he folded the napkin this way and that way as he tried to construct a hat origami-style. Part of me laughed as I watched him working so meticulously. But then I began to imagine Jack at fifteen and wondered, "Would he be the same?" Tears got the better of me, so off to the bathroom I went. Although Jack doesn't always pick up on other people's feelings, he is usually very sensitive to mine. I returned to the table to find Jack serenely eating the mussels; when I sat down, he looked up and said, "Thank you for at least not crying at the table."

Why was the origami experience so overwhelming for me? Because it made clear the amount of educating that I was facing. Not only did I have a child whom I had to specifically and repeatedly teach precise behavior lessons, I would also have to be at the ready to disengage hidden land mines. A typical child would have taken his learning on table manners and his learning about how to behave in public settings and probably would have behaved quite reasonably during dinner. In

Jack's case, I had to think through every aspect of the meal ahead of time – what would work for him, how he would react to the setting, the selection of foods offered, and even where the table was – and adjust them to fit his needs. And even with all this, I was hit broadside by an innocent remark.

This scenario taught me that it was not enough to see the world as Jack sees it so that I can anticipate what might occur and set up the environment with the greatest chance of success. I also had to be emotionally prepared for the unexpected, and be able to handle it with grace and humor, until the right time when I could address the issue with him.

You know more than you think you do about how your child views the world around him. You know a lot about how he takes in, processes, and understands information. Your child's diagnosis and symptoms provide clues. Some reflection based on how you see him operate will show you how much more you know. The exercise later in this chapter will help you think through how your child learns from the world.

In both restaurants I had taken careful pains to set up the environment and situation as best I could to accommodate how Jack sees and interacts with the world. The New York restaurant was a looser environment, but Jack was at a higher functioning level by then. In neither case, could I ultimately control how he thought and behaved, which was out of a perspective of doing what, first and foremost, felt comfortable to him and not thinking about the impact his behavior had on others.

I never went back to address the napkin situation with Jack. At that age and stage, I didn't think it would do any good. But the bread incident, I addressed head on because at that point he was ready to take some responsibility for his behavior and learn about self-control.

Two nights later I set up a very special dinner – our best china and silver and a gourmet meal, including some flaky, fresh-baked rolls. I asked my daughter to imitate what Jack had done at the New York restaurant, and to do so in a very low-key way, throughout the meal. We began the meal. Sarah started stuffing her face and overusing the butter. Halfway through the meal, I feigned horror and brought everyone's attention to her poor manners. Jack got the point. We had a good laugh over Sarah's performance. It wasn't until he literally *saw* the behavior right in front of him that Jack understood what others saw of him.

Why Do I Have to Do the Adjusting?

You have to do the adjusting because – at this stage – you can and your child can't. Don't get hung up on the apparent unfairness of the situation. It's reality. If you walk around angry that your child cannot see the forest or the trees, or anything else that seems so clear to you, you will get nowhere.

If you begin with knowing who your child is and how he thinks, how he processes and interprets information, you have a starting place for reaching him. As you are figuring out who this child is, you might see where his interpretation of the world can most easily be adjusted and where it is most important to do so. Over time, his cognitive and developmental growth will provide you with the necessary opening to begin to teach him how others see the world. When Jack says something that is beyond just a unique way of looking at something, I say to him, "It's fine for you to think that way with me but most boys your age would look at it like this …" And then I explain another viewpoint. Or I have someone else who works with Jack regularly show him the different viewpoint when the opportunity presents itself. Long term, you want to help your child shift his viewpoint but you can't do that until he has the cognitive ability and willingness to do so.

Applying Your Understanding of How Your Child Sees the World

When you are able to see the world through your child's eyes, you can use this information as a jumping-off point. Once you have a good handle on your child's temperament, how he is likely to react in situations, and how he will take in information and respond to it, you have quite a few tools with which to build those bridges. Here's an example of how it works.

Jack was doing math homework one night at 8 p.m. The math book introduced a new concept – using a calculator. Although I was already in my pajamas, Jack begged me to take him to Staples to buy a new calculator, since my calculator was not like the one in the book. "Fine," I agreed, thrilled that he was being so responsible with what was needed. "But I am ready for bed so should I change into clothes or can you get the calculator on your own?"

"No problem, I can handle it," he assured me, so off we went – Jack armed with twenty dollars and his book, me in nothing more than my fluffy pajamas and a coat. We got to the store and in Jack went to get the calculator. I waited and waited. At first, I rather liked the quiet of the car. It was restful and allowed me to catch a few winks.

But when those few minutes turned into forty-five minutes, I sighed, knowing that I had taken a risk, zipped my coat up as high as it would go, and shuffled into Staples. There was Jack, surrounded on the floor by every calculator type the store stocked. (Remember, he is very precise and exacting.) "Hey, Mom!" Jack shouted as soon as he saw me. "They don't have a calculator that is exactly like the one in my book!" I could have dealt with that. In fact, I was moving to deal with it. But then Jack added, in the loudest voice he had, "Mom, are you still wearing your pajamas?" And with that he bounced over and unzipped my coat to check for himself.

I had known there was a risk that Jack would somehow get hung up in the store. Usually he gets distracted from his mission and forgets the time or the fact that I am waiting in the car. I had thought to wear a coat just in case I needed to go in and get him. Just before he went in, I had reminded him what he was going in to get and gave him a slip of paper with the word calculator on it. What I had not anticipated (but saw the "logic" of the minute I walked in the store) was how exacting Jack would be in trying to find a calculator that matched the one he had seen in the book.

I used the situation to teach Jack. Quietly, I went over to a store manager and asked him to show Jack which calculator would do everything the one in the book did. I knew that having a store manager's opinion would hold a lot more weight than mine when it came to calculators. I was right. Jack accepted the store manager's recommendation. Jack was convinced that he had an acceptable calculator and, in the process, learned a little flexibility.

I was able to turn what could have been a disaster into something that taught a lesson because I could quickly assess the situation and see how my son was seeing the world. The more you get in tune with how your child sees things, the faster and more naturally you can avoid disasters and turn situations around. Whether it is enjoying a meal with friends or getting school supplies, teaching your child how to navigate these waters empowers him. They are the building blocks to navigating a larger world.

How Your Child Interprets the World Around Him

Understanding the differences in how children with special needs come to interpret their world will help you understand their behaviors and responses to what happens to them. Think about how your child learns from the world around him by doing the following exercise.

How Does Your Child Learn from the World?

	Yes	No	Sometimes
Picks up verbal cues	☐	☐	☐
Picks up nonverbal cues	☐	☐	☐
Listens to others	☐	☐	☐
Reads body language	☐	☐	☐
Makes eye contact	☐	☐	☐
Stays on topic	☐	☐	☐
Enjoys others' differences	☐	☐	☐
Notices others' differences	☐	☐	☐
Touches, smells, tastes	☐	☐	☐
Practices physically	☐	☐	☐
Rehearses verbally	☐	☐	☐
Takes apart	☐	☐	☐

Experiences Will Color How Your Child Sees the World

No one sees the world in a vacuum. As we grow and interact with the world, part of how we see it is based on the feedback that we receive. Many children with special needs get an enormous amount of negative feedback from the world on a variety of levels. As much as parents try to stay positive, we all have a limit, and our children are remarkably good at pushing it. Similarly, even the most patient of teachers can be pushed to her limits by the child who is constantly interrupting or creating havoc in the classroom. And the number of store clerks, innocent bystanders, and people you run into who think your kid is just plain "bad" and let him know it are more than you care to remember. All of these experiences affect your child and influence how he sees the world. Therefore, a large part of what you want to do once you understand how he sees the world is to help him better understand and negotiate the world at large.

A number of years ago, I was driving down our winding lane to pick Jack up from the bus stop the way I always do. He was already walking up the lane, hunkered down in his big, yellow ski jacket. As I drove up to him, he jumped in front of the car.

"Jack!" I yelled. "What are you doing?" If I had been driving any faster, I could easily have hit him. Jack came up to the window nonchalantly, unfazed by my upset.

"You didn't have a smile on your face. You looked bored," he said.

"So you decided to shake me up by jumping in front of the car?" I asked.

"Well, it worked, didn't it?" he replied.

Luckily, nothing bad had come of his impulsive move. And I knew, as he had said, that Jack saw the world for me as boring and wanted to find a solution. This was a perfect opportunity to explain what could have happened, and that sometimes it is okay to be a little bored. I must admit that I was more understanding than empathetic in that exchange.

Empathy. Patience. Short words but big concepts. Those concepts are what it takes to understand our children's views of the world around them. And when we understand their views, we can create a climate that is easier on them until the time when they can learn for themselves how to adjust their sights and do some adapting. For some children, that day is already here. Others may never be able to do more than what they are doing today. So for them, we must continue to do the adjusting.

So, here we are, hopefully with some clarity around your child's diagnosis and symptoms and then having put on a lens that allows us to see how the child views and interprets the world, given his uniqueness. That should be enough work to understand the child, right? Not exactly.

Say that your child is pretty impulsive, extremely hyper, and unfocused much of the time. He sees the world very often by catching just a piece of it because he is moving too quickly. One day, you plan a special treat to take him to a live performance of "The Lion King." You get to the theatre and are greeted in the lobby by some of the characters from the show – wonderful oversized animals of the jungle. Unexpectedly and surprisingly, your child pitches a tremendous fit. What's going on? You run through your mind all the symptoms of ADHD and try to see things how he is seeing them. Maybe the size of the theatre is too overwhelming for him. You ask the theatre attendant if you can sit on a side where your child won't feel the sense of a large crowd so intensely. But he continues to be fussy for the first half of the show, and when the intermission lights come on he tells you that he is not staying for the rest of the show. What happened? It all comes together the minute you start to look at "the inside child." The "inside child" is the last piece that will give you a comprehensive understanding of your child. Let's take a look at it next.

THE BOTTOM LINE

You have three goals in trying to understand how your child views the world:

- To make the world an easier place for him to negotiate and be successful by giving him tools and information to help him adjust to what he doesn't see or doesn't see fully or correctly.

- To anticipate and head off potential crises and problems.

- To know what impressions, attitudes, and interpretations will have to be adjusted, when the time is right.

CHAPTER 3

INSIDE THE BOX

Getting to Know What Doesn't Meet the Eye

The inside child consists of the things that are invisible to the eye but that drive your child's behaviors, shape his attitudes, and color the way in which he sees the world. Temperament, fears, passions, and feelings are examples of what makes up the inside child.

Knowing your child on the inside gives you information that can guide you in determining what needs to be worked on and how best to do so. Before we look at the inside child, let's see how well you know the child in general.

HOW WELL DO YOU KNOW YOUR CHILD?

You might think that you know him well. Maybe that is because you spend a lot of time together. However, we can spend a lot of time with someone and still not really know who the person is.

Test yourself. See how easily you can complete the following exercise. After you fill out the first half, check out your answers with your child to see if you were on target.

THINKING INSIDE THE BOX

1. What is your child's greatest passion? _____
2. What are two fears of your child? _____
3. What does your child think he is incompetent at? _____
4 What does your child think he is competent at? _____
5. Does your child see his cup as half empty or half full? _____

Write "T" next to the statements below that you believe are true. If you are unsure, put the letter "U" next to the statement.

1. My child is self-absorbed. _____
2. My child is sensitive to the feelings of others. _____
3. My child doesn't understand when he hurts others. _____
4. My child is a concrete thinker. _____

Maybe it was easy for you to do the exercise *and* you are fairly confident that you were on target, but here's the million-dollar question: "How do you know that your responses were accurate?" Before you congratulate yourself, perhaps you want to think about "testing" your hypotheses. You might do this by asking others who work with your child to complete the exercise as well.

If, on the other hand, you were scratching your head in trying to come up with answers to the exercise, perhaps a little more getting to know your child, the inside of your child, is in order.

BUILDING ON STRENGTHS

All children possess attributes that make them feel accomplished and that they are good at something. These strengths and abilities, which Drs. Robert Brooks and Sam Goldstein call "islands of competence,"[10] are what give a child a sense of purpose and make him feel successful. Islands of competence are not always obvious. They may be as subtle as having a warm personality or demonstrating strong endurance. As a parent interested in helping your child along his path, it is important that you identify and draw on your child's islands of competence.

---

[10] *Raising Resilient Children* (New York: McGraw-Hill, 2001).

Recognizing your child's competencies gives you a place to build from. When Jack was two and a half years old with minimal language, the speech therapist hooked into what has remained one of his islands – a deep knowledge of nature and animals. She bought a deck of animal cards filled with information and used them as a springboard to work on his speech and language goals. Jack thought he was becoming a naturalist, but in reality, the speech therapist was doing what was necessary to get done what he was otherwise unmotivated to do.

There once lived a boy who learned by doing. At the age of six, he wanted to see how fire worked and burned his father's barn down to the ground. The next fall, and not a moment too soon, the boy began his formal schooling.

"Good," thought his parents. "This will keep Tom's young mind busy."

School did not go well for Tom. The boy was distracted and restless, making it difficult for the teacher to keep control of the class. Before long, the school asked Tom's parents to remove him. Years later, Tom recalled this time in his life: "My father thought I was stupid, and I almost decided to be a dunce."

But Tom's mother had other ideas for her son and set to home-schooling the boy. Tom's mother knew her son had a passion for experiments, and as his new teacher she encouraged this interest. At the same time, she fostered a sense of discipline in him. With the determination of both mother and son, Tom learned how to control his spirited mind.

The boy who grew up to be an inventor, bringing the birth of electricity, sound recovery, and hundreds of everyday conveniences to the world, was none other than Thomas Edison.[11]

This story is the perfect example of drawing on a child's competencies rather than focusing on his weaknesses. You can easily imagine a different scenario. One where Tom is asked to leave school and his parents take a punitive approach. Maybe they make him work in the fields or put him in a school that will "straighten him out." Using one of Tom's strengths to work on a deficit was a brilliant move by Mrs. Edison. She didn't have to beg, cajole, or threaten her son to get his act together. In captivating his interest and linking his love of science with developing a disciplined mind, she also offered him an opportunity to further his talents.

---

[11] Lucy Jo Palladino, *The Edison Trait* (New York: Times Books, 1997).

Someone once asked Thomas Edison how he felt about all of his failed experiments. He said he had no failed experiments. It just took him two thousand and one tries to get it right – seems he was also able to develop a positive attitude toward the whole process.

I should note that there is a thin line for some children between passions and obsessions. A passion has crossed over to being an obsession when it interferes with healthy daily functioning. This can be particularly true for children with Asperger Syndrome or obsessive/compulsive disorder (OCD). Draw on your child's strengths and passions. But remember, they should be used to broaden the child, not to define him.

IDENTIFY LIMITING THOUGHTS, FEELINGS, AND ATTITUDES

It is as important to identify what things inside the child may be contributing to negative behaviors as it is to identify the strengths, interests, and passions you should play to. For the sake of language, let's call these negative things "prickly parts." Here's an example.

For the longest time I thought that Jack had no sensitivity. No feelings for anyone. But over time, I learned that he was actually hypersensitive, with many fears and an overactive imagination to boot. What looked like negative behaviors was often Jack being afraid or oversensitive.

Knowing the parts of your child's temperament, thoughts, and emotions that result in negative feelings and behaviors can help you anticipate and head off problems. These are also areas that most likely should be worked on. Keeping your head in the sand and pretending that they will take care of themselves does no good. Changing your child may seem impossible, but helping him to recognize who he is and how he comes across is a first step toward what later can be his choice to focus on.

Knowing what the prickly parts are is very helpful in determining how you interact with your child, and they should be taken into consideration when you establish his goals.

GETTING TO THE INSIDE CHILD

Your child's personality is what it is. You will never be able (or want) to fundamentally change his temperament (his self-set).[12] However, the more you understand your child's self-set, along with his heart-set and mind-set, the more you will

[12]   Robin Kencel and Sally Eberhardt, *I Only Have a Minute So This Better Be Good* (Greenwich, CT: Publication pending).

be able to develop a Life Map that will be appropriate for him, and the more you will know what you and others who work with him have to pay attention to.

Getting inside somebody is easier said than done. You can't just sit down and ask, "So, what's going on in your inside? Tell me about your interests, your fears, what you like, and what you hate." You especially can't do this with a preteen or teenager. Being around, being available, but not in your child's face, is the only way that you are going to see what is not on the surface.

Step back for a minute and take a look at yesterday's interactions with your child. Answer the following questions and think for a minute about how you feel about your answers.

Are You Connecting to the Inside Child?

1. How many minutes did you spend engaged in conversation with your child yesterday? _____

2. During that time, were you you-focused or him-focused? _____

3. Do you understand your child as well as you would like to? _____

Spending a few minutes at bedtime, sitting on the bed and asking your child how his day was, is often a good way to get to know him at this deeper level. For some reason, when children are comfortably nestled under the covers, they seem to be less resistant and more willing to share what is inside. The car is another good place to open up conversation. This is where Jack and I had "the talk." It started out routinely enough at the pick-up line outside of school. Jack was in fourth grade.

"Mom, some kids were talking about 'it,'" he started. I knew exactly what he meant. If this conversation had taken place at home, any number of things could have prevented it from continuing. More than likely, something would have caught Jack's eye and distracted him, and that would have been the end of it. But in the car, free from anything that could interrupt, I could explain the "birds and the bees" to him. Just enough information to answer the follow-up questions and to cover what I thought he might hear from his peers. Then when we got home, I took out the book I had been storing, *What's Going On Down There? Answers to Questions Boys Find Difficult to Ask,*[13] a book for boys on puberty that is written

[13] Karen Gravelle et al. (New York: Walker Publishing Company, 1998).

with a humorous but appropriate tone that I had thought would keep his interest and give him the facts of growing up – from the need for underarm deodorant as he hit his teens to how his body would be changing.

For us, the car seems to be the place where we cover these sorts of big-deal issues and have our deeper-level discussions. You will find a place and time that suits you and your child best. Get to know your child's rhythms (Is he a morning person or a night owl? When is he most open to conversation?) and where he is most comfortable.

THE BOTTOM LINE

- The inside child is what lies beneath outward behaviors and perspectives. It is your child's unique mix of temperament, attitudes, emotions, and thoughts.

- Using a strength-based approach – that is, drawing on your child's interests, passions, and strengths – develops a sense of capability and feelings of self-worth in your child.

- Identifying the thoughts, feelings, and attitudes that limit the child is as important as acknowledging his strengths.

- The more time you invest to understand your child, the easier your journey with him will be.

- When you are oriented to and interested in knowing the inside of your child, you will find the ways to best reach him. Once you are in the right listening mode, you will hear the things that are under the surface.

CHAPTER 4

WHERE DOES THE CHILD FIT IN?

The Path to Self-Understanding

Although this section has focused on all the ways in which you can reach out to your child and meet him where he is, the eventual goal is for your child to be able to adapt to the world around him. Based upon his own limitations and strengths, he will be able to do this to a greater or lesser degree. Your role in moving him towards self-awareness and responsibility and taking the lead in his own growth and development is to be the support and guidance that he will need as he moves from your being in the control seat to his being there. Just as you have to understand him, he has to understand himself.

Being self-reflective and able to look with an objective eye at your own actions, as well as the actions of those you interact with, is not automatic for many people. If you are someone who is objective, intuitive, and introspective, you might be able to provide the guidance that your child needs to grow in this area. This is a tall order for some of us. Take a look at professionals – perhaps the social worker or psychologist at your child's school, a teacher or a coach – and see who in your child's life might make some inroads in helping him develop this self-awareness, when opportunities present themselves.

Jack's sixth-grade teachers were wonderful at playing this role for him. When an incident came up with another student or an adult, Jack's teachers always sat down with him and worked through the issues, making him take responsibility for the situation, when appropriate, and learn to understand his role in it and what he could have done differently. Although Jack often went through the motions of correcting the situation begrudgingly, he began to understand how others' thoughts and feelings – and how different they could be from his own. For example, Jack's frequent retort, "I thought it was funny!" when he said something insulting to a classmate was not always viewed as being funny by the recipient of the comment. If no one had taken the time to explain and help Jack see a different viewpoint, and give him the opportunity to practice making his wrong, right, he might never have shifted his understanding of what is appropriate humor.

You and those who work with your child will know how much and how fast you can work on developing his self-awareness. Don't try to push him beyond what he is capable of. All you will do is frustrate yourself and him. Remember, your child's life is a process that has its own rhythm and timing. Work with it.

THE BOTTOM LINE

- Understanding your child is step one. Helping your child understand himself is step two.

- Your child will eventually need to develop self-awareness to monitor his own actions and behaviors so that he can make the right choices. Since self-awareness probably doesn't come naturally to him, you (or competent people you put in his path) will be an important part of teaching him this skill.

- Regardless of where your child is in his emotional and cognitive maturity, you can still plant seeds, appropriate to his current developmental level, that will begin the process of unfolding his tent towards understanding who he is underneath.

SECTION 2

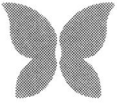

UNDERSTANDING YOURSELF

CHAPTER 1

THREE SETS, ANYONE?
Self-Set, Heart-Set and Mind-Set

In a national longitudinal study conducted in 1996-97,[14] researchers sought to identify what were the most important variables that prevented teens from becoming at risk. The study interviewed 14,000 teens, aged fourteen to nineteen. Results showed that the number-one factor was the teens' sense of connectedness to their mother and/or father. *Connectedness* meant feeling valued, accepted, loved, and supported. The second most important factor was a feeling of being connected at school; that is, being accepted and valued and having positive relationships with teachers and peers.

Most likely, the majority of parents know on some level how significant their impact is on their children's lives. So why do we sometimes behave in ways that are not supportive, encouraging, or even particularly kind? I suspect that if we could pull back from the situation and watch a tape of how we are behaving, we would often change what we are doing.

---

[14] "Adolescent Well-Being in Cohabiting, Married, and Single-Parent Families," Wendy D. Manning, *American Journal of Marriage and Family,* 65(4), November, 2003.

Sarah, our daughter, is thirteen, and Jack is now eleven. Both children have emerged in the last year or so as parent police officers.

"What's with your tone, Mom?" Jack will ask as I tell him for the twentieth time to hang up his coat and put away his shoes after he bursts through the door from school.

"That sounds snippy!" Sarah will say in the middle of one of our battles about curfew, bedtime, or what kind of makeup (if any) she is allowed to wear.

Lately, I have begun to listen to myself as I am speaking to my children – or rather, when I am in a heated discussion, which is when the unattractive tones usually appear. I have learned a lot by doing this. For starters, that I don't always act in ways that are consistent with what I believe is the right way, that I sometimes have a rather negative spin on my kids, and that, to be completely honest, I occasionally don't like them very much.

What determines who we are and how we respond to the people and events in our life are three basics:

- **S E L F - S E T** – The traits, temperament, and characteristics that we come into the world with.

- **H E A R T - S E T** – The feelings that we have towards ourselves and others.

- **M I N D - S E T** – Our attitudes and perceptions.

Knowing yourself and how these three work inside of you is essential if you want to be more in control of your actions, feelings, and outlook. And one of the most important ways to do this is to be self-aware. This section takes a closer look at the three "sets" and how they can impact your actions and your relationships with others.

Incidentally, understanding how these fundamentals play out in your child is important. The child's disorder and disabilities, along with the particular personality and character temperament that he was born with, are part of his *self-set*. The inside child, how he feels about things, is part of his *heart-set*. And how the child sees the world is his beginning steps toward developing attitudes and perceptions, or his *mind-set*.

SELF-SET

The self-set is the fundamental that you have the least control over. What falls into the self-set is the part that is your "nature" – that is, the genetic mix that made you who you are. Your self-set is largely influenced by two factors – your temperament and the impact that your own family had on you as you grew up.

TEMPERAMENT

Just as your child was born with a specific temperament and character traits, so were you. Suppose you were born incredibly shy. You were the one in elementary school who never spoke out. You had just one good friend. People thought you were nice, but you rarely said anything so they didn't know you well. One day, you decide that you are tired of being shy. You enroll in a Dale Carnegie course and change your style to show real personality. And, sure enough, you do become a little less shy. But you don't become Ms. Gregarious. It just isn't in your nature. You've moved the dial of shyness, but in the end, shyness is still a part of you because it is part of your biological makeup.

The degree to which you can change a character trait, if you want to, depends on what the trait is, how deeply engrained it is, how hard you are willing to work at it, and how much you want to change. For example, if you were born cranky, the kind of person who tends to whine the moment anything goes wrong, you aren't stuck with that persona. Training yourself to say, "Now where do I see the goodness in that?" and "What went well in my life today?" can begin to alter the way you respond to life.

Your temperament influences how you interact with your child, and these interactions can have a huge impact on him. Examine how your specific traits affect your relationship with your child by filling in the following exercise.

THE GOOD, THE BAD, AND THE HERE TO STAY

- Name one character trait of yours that you believe positively contributes to your relationship with your child. _____

- Name one character trait of yours that you believe negatively impacts your relationship with your child. _____

ROLE OF FAMILY

There are many elements of your own family that have influenced who you are and impacted how you parent. The three major factors are your parents' parenting style, your birth order, and your siblings. Taking a little time to think about how these each played a role in developing who you are will help you determine how you are relating to others and particularly to your child.

Parenting Style

Depending on how you felt about your parents, you have gone on to either reject or emulate how they parented you. But whatever style you have adopted may or may not work with the type of child you have. For example, if you are a tense, tightly strung person and you have a cranky baby, chances are the two of you will be butting heads. If you are more relaxed and calm, you are probably better equipped to handle the strain of a baby who is whiny and demanding. The child is not going to change his style to suit you. You will have to adjust yourself by adopting a parenting style that works for him. See how well you know your own style and how you think it fits with your child.

DOES YOUR PARENTING STYLE FIT YOUR CHILD'S NEEDS?

How would you describe your child's general temperament?

_____

_____

How would you describe your parenting style, thinking about your own temperament?

_____

_____

What are two things that you think you could do differently in your style that would make a positive impact on your parenting?

1. _____

2. _____

Birth Order

You are also affected by where you were in your family's birth order. There are general characteristics associated with each position in the family: firstborn, middle, youngest, and only child. Firstborns can be perfectionists, headstrong, high achievers, goal driven, well organized, and conscientious.[15] This is partly due to

---

[15] Kevin Leman, *The New Birth Order Book* (Grand Rapids, MI: Baker Book House Co., 1998); Meri Wallace, *Birth Order Blues* (New York: Henry Bolt and Co., 1989).

all the attention and expectations put upon them as the first child in the family. Only children are similar to firstborns; however, they can be a bit self-centered if they have not had enough exposure to peers.

Middle children are often independent, good at thinking on their feet, resilient, and gregarious. Feeling like they have no special place in the family, they look for attention from friends and the outside world. They are good mediators. Generally speaking, being middle-born is a good position to come from as a parent of a child with special needs. They know how to get things done, but are flexible about how they do them. They are good at drawing people together and getting them involved, which is important in creating the team that will be needed to support the child.

The youngest siblings are known for having easygoing personalities, with an almost "devil-may-care" attitude. They may the entertainers and play upon all the extra attention that they got as the baby of the family. This is not always a good place to come from if you are a parent of a child with special needs. If you are a youngest, you may have to pull up your bootstraps and realize that if you go with the flow, you could end up anywhere.

Siblings
Your experience with your siblings was your first exposure to peer social skills. In the process you learned all sorts of social skills lessons – sharing, negotiating, learning to live with differences, resolving conflict, and more. How your parents managed your sibling squabbles and nurtured your family unit impacted how you think about the family. Being a little aware of what the major dynamics were will give you insight into how you may be going about your own parenting.

Once you understand your self-set and how your temperament and family are part of you, you are better prepared to parent your own child.

HEART-SET
Heart-set is about your feelings. The heart-set you have toward each person in your life is different and often changing. Your children, your spouse, your friends, and those you work with all elicit different reactions and emotions. You also have a heart-set toward yourself.

For many of us, our feelings toward our exceptional child are very complex. We know that we should love this child, but honestly, from the minute he gets up until he goes to bed, he can drive us crazy. I always marvel at how *nice* a person I can be all day long until four o'clock in the afternoon. Within five minutes of my son walking through the door after school, I can become completely undone.

Love him? Like him? Not always possible. It has been said, "Children who are in need of the greatest love ask for it in the most unlovable ways." Children with challenging behaviors are masterful at pushing the wrong buttons, either by what they do or by what they don't do (but are supposed to be doing).

There are times, if we are completely honest with ourselves, where anger seems to be the feeling of the day. The problem with anger is that it is such a strong feeling that it overpowers love. I may love my child, but when I am angry I can't feel much of anything besides that anger and all the horrible things that go along with it. Negative feelings can overcome your rational thinking and logic. Being aware of how you are feeling is a first step in keeping your emotions in check.

Take some time to think about how you honestly feel about your child. Complete the following exercise to get a sense of where your feelings are.

I FEEL SO MIXED UP

What was my child doing the last time I felt:

sad	_____	happy	_____
proud	_____	excited	_____
annoyed	_____	lonely	_____

You may have a heart-set toward your child that seems to be punctuated by anger, dislike, or other unpleasant feelings much of the time. That is understandable. Do not feel guilty about your feelings. But don't just sit there with them either.

How you feel about your child often translates into how you treat him. According to educators and consultants who work with exceptional children, it appears that many children see the adults around them as negative and not believing in them. This in turn can negatively affect their performance and influence their actions. If you want your child to feel good about himself, he needs to know that you believe he can make it. Much of this is conveyed through the way you make him feel. Do you focus on the positive things he accomplishes? Or do you keep a list of negative behaviors and issues at your fingertips, ready to point to them at the first sign of trouble?

The standard you should be holding yourself to is respect. I am constantly reminding my children to respect others, so I should speak to them in a tone and manner that is respectful. My children deserve the same respect that I ask them to show and that I show to everyone else.

It is difficult to fake your feelings. You might think you can pretend to be warm and loving on the outside while disappointment and anger prowl around inside, but that doesn't hold up in the long run. Putting on a front won't fool anyone, not even a child who otherwise isn't the best at reading social cues. Whether it's your child, your spouse, the team, or a friend, it is best to face the feelings that are creating barriers so that you can move forward.

As children, my siblings and I knew that our mother's most important and meaning-ful possession was her Hummel collection. She had over fifty of these wonderful porce-lain figurines, which she proudly displayed on the bookshelves in our family room. Like a Norman Rockwell painting, each one portrayed a different sliver of a child's life. Every figurine had been given to my mother by us children, my father, or other close relatives. She was known for her collection and held it near and dear to her heart.

One evening I was enmeshed in homework and raced down to the family room to look up something in the World Book encyclopedia. The encyclopedia was on a book-shelf held in place by wonderful Hummel bookends. With mind and hands moving too fast, I pulled a book from the shelf and with it, the Hummel bookend! I held my breath as I picked up the figurine. It came up in one piece. That was the good news. As I inspected it more closely, however, I noticed that one of the hands of the seated child had broken off. I scooped up the hand that lay nearby, pocketed it, and moved the bookend to the far side so the missing hand would be against the back of the book-shelf. I hoped my mother wouldn't notice.

As each day passed, a little thread of panic and fear grew around my heart as I waited to see if my mother would notice what had happened to one of the most important pieces of her collection. My worry grew as Tuesday neared. Tuesday was her major cleaning day and the day that all of the Hummels were taken down from the shelves to be dusted.

But several weeks went by with no discovery of my accident. I stayed busy and kept a good distance from my mother. I was so afraid that if she read my eyes she would discover my secret. Ironically, on Good Friday, nearly two months after the mishap, my mother discovered what had happened. She had enlisted my sister's and my help for a top-to-bottom cleaning in preparation for Easter dinner with our relatives.

"Does anyone know how this happened?" my mother asked, looking at the disfigured Hummel she had picked up to dust. I looked at her blankly, as did my sister. No one said a word. My mother wrapped it carefully in tissue paper and tucked it away in a closet. It wasn't mentioned again.

I couldn't sleep that night. I felt horrible for not being honest with my mother, on top of being exhausted from two months of worry and fear. That chipped Hummel had somehow wedged a distance between my mother and me. Anxious, I got out of bed and found her ironing in the kitchen.

My mother didn't scold me or yell at me when I told her what I had done. I remember what she said: "It is more important that you told me the truth than anything else. Accidents happen, but maybe this will teach you that you need to slow down a little." My heart was lifted miles high that night. The awful feelings that had distanced me from my mother dissolved. She had forgiven me instantly, and done so in the most gentle of ways. I never forgot that Hummel.

What the Hummel experience taught me was how powerful feelings are in relationships. I couldn't believe how negative my feelings had become toward my mother, what with my worrying and my fear of how she would react to what I had done. And I couldn't believe how my feelings toward myself had changed as well.

YOU HAVE FEELINGS, EVEN ABOUT YOURSELF

How you feel about yourself is not always easy to figure out, nor is it easy to determine how you came to feel that way. Our feelings about ourselves come from a variety of places. Perhaps the most important sources are how others treat us, particularly how our parents treated us and made us feel when we were young, and what happened in our past. Sometimes all it takes is one solid positive relationship for our world to turn right-side up, or one bad relationship or experience for the trajectory of how we feel about ourselves to turn negative forever.

Many of us tend to focus on the worst side or moments of our lives. At the end of the day, do you say to yourself, "Hey, self, that was a nice job you did today listening to other people's ideas in the meeting and not shutting them off," or do you start rehashing things that you wish you had handled differently? Mistakes and slip-ups are inevitable. Who among us can avoid thinking about how we hurt a friend, wounded a child, shipwrecked a relationship, or much worse? What we do with these negative experiences, in terms of how we absorb them into our own life, impacts how we feel and think about ourselves.

As the parent of a child with special needs, your odds of making errors go way up, which means opportunities to see yourself as a failure or having failed increase as well. That is because your situation demands much higher virtue-like abilities in almost battle-like conditions. Mistakes are bound to happen in greater proportion when you're placed in such a high-stress setting, particularly in the early years when you are unclear about what your child's issues are and have little training or preparation to deal with them.

How you respond to what you have done, or not done, boomerangs and affects how you feel and think about yourself. Saying, "I am a failure," is very different from saying, "I made a mistake." The first statement you use to define yourself – and that can be limiting – and the second you use to learn from. Your view of your mistakes is only one strand in a ball of yarn that makes up who you are and how you see yourself. The greater your self-awareness and understanding of who you are, the more you will be able to take your experiences – mistakes and all – and study them and learn from them. And that will influence, in a positive way, how you feel and think about yourself.

KNOW WHAT YOU ARE FEELING

"How is Jack doing?" friends and acquaintances ask.
"Great," I say, lying through my teeth.

Maybe you are the kind of person who says what you think people want to hear. Maybe you don't feel like sharing the underside of the rug. Or maybe you are too worn out to keep repeating yourself so you say what they want to hear or what you think is best to say. But it's wearing, and perhaps untrue. And maybe it's not just those around you that you are lying to. You might be lying to yourself as well.

Or maybe you are the type of person who is constantly complaining, telling everyone about your troubles. Although this gives you a little relief at the moment, in the end you still feel the same: not good.

How about trying something completely different? How about focusing on the *good* qualities? When Sarah became a teen, it was just as my friends with older daughters had warned me: good-bye "nice" (to me anyway), hello "attitude."

Luckily for me, at the time I was writing a general self-help book with Sally, the amazing psychotherapist. It is just a coincidence that Sally and I do some of our brainstorming at my house, and I get to see her in action with my children. Direct, on-the-spot training.

One of the things that Sally has taught me is to look at Sarah's gifts rather than focusing on what I think she "should" be. The more I harped on grades and manners, grades and manners, the more the two slipped away. One day Sally said, "If you would just work on enjoying Sarah and worry less, you would see a whole different girl. She really is quite terrific."

That same week, through a fluke connection, a magazine asked Sarah and me to be part of a holiday fashion spread of mothers and daughters. The mothers were to wear an outfit one way, and the daughters, a completely different way. Since my daughter wanted nothing to do with being like me, I wasn't sure how this would play out. But she is very interested in fashion and was all for the shoot.

I went into the day with the heart-set that Sally had suggested. Through the editor's and photographer's eyes and accolades, I saw a young lady who was inquisitive, poised, and spirited. She radiated the entire day. At the end of the shoot, the editor said to me, "It's a little frightening that she knows so much about fashion, but she is also incredibly well grounded. You've done a great job with her." To Sarah she said, "Call me in about four years. You would make a great candidate for an internship." From that day forward, I have tried to look at least as much at the positive as the negative with Sarah. And it has affected both our heart-sets.

Regardless of whether what you say is positive or negative, knowing what you feel is an important part of understanding how you relate to your child. For those feelings toward your child that are not so hot, you'll want to try to change. First things first. Let's take a look at how you feel about working on this stuff.

Working on My Feelings

Check the statement that best reflects your thoughts on your feelings:

_____ My feelings are fine. Next question.

_____ I guess I need to do some work on my feelings.

_____ I've been waiting for someone to ask me how I feel. Let's get to work!

If you checked the second or third statement, you're ready for the next exercise. However, if you checked the first statement, you are best off doing some thinking about why you don't want to look more closely at this issue. Remember, you are in the driver's seat here. You don't have to change anything – including your feelings – that you don't want to. But if you open yourself up a little, you may find that you want to make a few adjustments.

If you are having negative feelings toward your child, it is good if you can be a little more precise in defining what they are. Take a minute and write down the feelings that come to mind when you think about your child. Here are a few words to help you get started. Feel free to circle as many of the words that reflect how you typically feel.

My Feelings About My Child

Angry	Sorry	Unforgiving
Frustrated	Disgusted	Judgmental
Hate	Embarrassed	Worried
Mad	Heartless	Proud
Exasperated	Joyless	Supportive
Impatient	Intolerant	Loving

There is a better way to manage than just letting the negative feelings overcome you. If you take the time and pay attention to the feelings you are experiencing as you go through your day and as you spend time with your child, you have made some solid progress. Knowing your feelings is a good start. The next step is to learn how to shift the negative ones, even if just a little.

TAKE CHARGE OF YOUR FEELINGS

Frustration, disappointment, anger, and confusion are common feelings when dealing with the often overwhelming challenges that come with raising a child with special needs. It is important that you acknowledge what you are feeling, but that does not mean you have to be a slave to your feelings. You have the power to change them.

Taking charge of each situation by getting beyond what is causing the negative feelings and finding something positive is a critical step toward changing your heart-set. Feelings can drive not only the way you feel about a person but how you think of him as well. The thinking domain is what the next section, the mind-set, is all about.

MIND-SET

When attitudes and perceptions become fixed, they become your mind-set, which decides ahead of time what your responses to, and interpretations of, a person or situation will be. Your perspective influences everything – your reactions at the moment, how you view your situation, your energy level, your happiness quotient, and your decision-making process. The following example illustrates this point.

Mrs. Miller is a fourth-grade teacher at Ramsey Elementary School. It is the first day of school. Mrs. Miller walks into her class and is soundly hit on the side of her face by a spitball. She looks around the room. In the first seat in the first row is Anthony Ferrell. Or rather, "Animal Anthony," as the teachers call him. "Anthony," Mrs. Miller says as she walks up to him. "Stop with the spit balls. I am not going to put up with those kinds of antics this year." Anthony looks up from the comic book he is reading, oblivious to what Mrs. Miller is talking about.

Mrs. Miller sure had a strong opinion for only 8:45 in the morning – and on the first day of school at that! Why did she come down so hard on Anthony?

Mrs. Miller had a negative mind-set toward Anthony before she even saw him in the classroom. Based on what she had heard from teachers Anthony had had in the past, she assumed he was going to behave a certain way before he even walked in. He didn't have to do (or not do) a single thing. He was a marked man because of her mind-set about him. Mrs. Miller was working off of a mind-set that said, "This kid is trouble, and I'm going to let him know who is boss right from the get-go." Her perception was that he was going to be a behavioral problem.

Take a moment to think about your mind-set toward your child and complete the following exercise.

What Is Your Mind-Set?

Write down a sentence or two that describe your attitudes, perceptions, and disposition toward your child. Try to think in terms of how you see your child, not just how you feel about him.

_____

_____

_____

_____

_____

LIMIT YOUR NEGATIVE THOUGHTS

Sometimes we get comfortable in the negative mode. We find ourselves telling anyone who is willing to listen how difficult our life is. We share the drama of what our child did today – or yesterday, the day before, or the day before that. There is never a lack of material to draw from, and we are happy to dish it out for all to hear. The way you think about your child impacts how you relate to him and how you present him to others. The more you let yourself think negatively, the more you will be negative with him and talk negatively about him. It becomes a vicious circle.

This is not to say that you should keep what you think to yourself. With your spouse, close friends, or a professional (such as a mental health professional), it is important to let your guard down and share what is on your mind. You need comfort, support, and other viewpoints besides your own every step of the way. Letting your hair down should be done very discriminately and not obsessively. Too much is the point where you go from letting it out so that you can move on to overthinking, overacting, and overdoing how you feel and think. Only you can determine what this point is. Being conscious of how much – and what – you are talking and thinking about your child is a first step toward determining if you are in a balanced state or not.

IT OFTEN STARTS OUT AS A FOOTNOTE

A number of factors influence your mind-set. Often, an attitude or perception starts out as a footnote – a small acknowledgment of something that happened that forms an impression about a person in your mind. At first, you are on your toes to see if this is a one-shot deal or if there is something more. You keep an eye out, and maybe the thing that caught your eye becomes an opinion. You "try it on," so to speak, and before you know it, a mind-set has developed.

You go out to dinner at Lucibello's Pizzeria with your friend, who is nasty to the waiter all evening. You haven't seen this side of her before, and you are not impressed. Maybe she is just having a bad day. You would hate to think that she is the kind of person whose kindness is situational. You tuck the experience away and don't think much about it.

A few weeks go by and you and this same friend go out for a day of shopping. As the day progresses, you notice that your friend is a little impatient with the salesclerks, demanding rather than asking for different sizes and such. The light bulb goes off and you remember what happened at Lucibello's. It all comes tumbling back. You start to form a full-blown opinion: Your friend is only nice to the people whom she wants to be nice to.

Now your antennae are up, and you see more signs that your opinion is correct. Now you have an out-and-out perception of your friend. It has become part of your mind-set.

WHAT DRIVES YOUR MIND-SET?

Attitudes and perceptions don't develop from nothing. Several factors can influence and feed their growth. Being aware of what these might be can help you to understand how your attitudes and perceptions got to where they are.

Fears and Insecurities

George is a twelve-year-old boy who was diagnosed as having pervasive developmental disabilities (PDD) when he was four. He worked closely with a speech and language pathologist for years and is on medication to treat low-grade, generalized anxiety. He is a brilliant student and a solid hockey, soccer, and lacrosse player.

George is on several travel teams, where he is not the star athlete but certainly not the worst either. In the car after every game, George's father thoroughly and completely reviews the game, detailing what his son could have done better and what he should work on for next time. By the end of the ride home, George doesn't feel very good about himself.

I stood next to George's father at a soccer game one day and listened firsthand to his running commentary on his son. In an effort to understand his negative tack with his son, I asked this dad what sports he had played as a kid and beyond. "None," he answered brusquely. "I had to help my father in his shoe store after school every day so I never had a chance to play any sport, and by the time I got to high school I was too far behind the other kids to be on the team."

That account explained the father's harshness with his son. He was trying to make George into the athlete that he had never had an opportunity to be himself. Fear and insecurity were driving his behavior. Unfortunately, he couldn't see beyond his mind-set.

Expectations and Dreams
My husband was looking forward to a second child. He had grown up with no siblings in a household where both his parents passed away at unusually early ages. He had so many dreams of what he would do as a father. Unfortunately, his long list of what he wanted, what he would do, and how he would act, completely fell apart when he had a son who could not connect to him one iota in the beginning.

John was disappointed with the cards life had dealt him in terms of his son. The two were at such odds with each other, Jack doing his own thing and John trying to get Jack to do the typical thing, that the relationship was in shambles by the time Jack was seven.

We brought a family therapist into the picture. The therapist worked with John to help him see that he could indeed have a relationship with his son, and a good one at that. It just wouldn't be the one that he had expected or dreamed about. Once John was able to let go of his expectations, he found that he did have places and ways to connect with Jack.

Today, the two could not be closer. In fact, just last week when Jack was tired of me "suggesting" that he move at a faster clip to get to a sports lesson, he turned around at the door and said,

"Send Dad to pick me up. He's a lot nicer and much cooler."

Granted, Jack was mad at me, but even if he wasn't, I think he now sees John as the one he connects with the best. John has mastered the art of seeing the cup as half full and reminds me at times when I have just about drained the cup of how much we have to be thankful for. When I ask him if he isn't just a little disappointed with how things turned out, he answers, "Are you kidding? I thought I'd never even *have* a son. I thought he would never relate to me. He's come so far. He's terrific! I'll take what we've got in a heartbeat."

At every stage of my life as a mother, I have expectations. I have expectations of what our family should be like, what I should be like, and what my husband and children should be like. Because I grew up on "Father Knows Best," "My Three Sons," and "The Donna Reed Show," my vision often looks like a mix of these television families. But when a parent holds a concrete expectation of how the family should be, a teacher has an ideal classroom in mind, or a therapist wishes for the perfect therapy session, it signals a set-up for failure.

Nothing is ever perfect; few things go according to plan. So holding on to expectations doesn't do much more than frustrate you and put undue pressure on your child.

Sports start at an early age in our town. Three years old to be exact. It's the talk of Saturday night dinner parties and after-church chitchat – how your child's team did and which fields you were going to and from for the balance of the weekend.

In theory, town sports sounded like a pretty good option for Jack. He could work on his eye-hand coordination and overall motor planning deficiencies. He could work on his social skills as well. We signed Jack up for fall baseball. We spoke with both the director and his coach, and were ready to go. That is, we were ready, but Jack wasn't. When he was three, it was the butterflies, at four it was chasing field crickets, at five it was picking dandelions, and when he was six, it was all three.

Clearly, he was not ready for team sports. Having a first-grade baseball dropout might seem like nothing to most, but in our New England town every sports field is filled on Saturday and Sunday. One of a parent's greatest thrills is having his child make the cut on whatever travel sport is in season. All those recent articles about overenthusiastic sports parents are written for a reason – parents are very invested in their kids' sports.

After the last disaster, we sat out a few seasons and regrouped in second grade. The start was rocky; Jack did not want to play the position the coach assigned him to. Unfortunately, he made that determination in the middle of a game and quit then and there. Third grade brought more drama. Jack declared himself a switch hitter. The coach tolerated two strikeouts before asking Jack to return to his right-handed batting position, which was already enough of a challenge for him. Jack dropped the bat and left the field. Game – and season – over.

What was up with this kid? "We've been through this quitting thing too many times," I said to Jack driving home from the game, tears streaming down my face. At his age, I was desperate to have him do what "normal" boys do. I knew from having two brothers that, for most boys, sports were how they connected to each other, what they talked about, and what they dreamed of. How was Jack ever going to fit in?

I was mad. I had done a great deal of homework to make baseball work for Jack that year. I finally had figured out the special-needs thing, or so I thought. The league director had made sure that we had a coach skilled with kids like Jack; I had hired a high school baseball star, who had worked for weeks to get Jack's skills up to par; and I had sat through every practice and game in case some on-site issue came up that Jack couldn't manage on his own. All this preparation and it still didn't work.

Jack stopped sniffling long enough to whisper into his shirt loud enough for me to hear, "I don't like baseball. It's your thing."

I had never thought about that. I had prided myself on making sure that everything was set up for Jack to succeed, but I had forgotten one thing. And it was the most important: Jack's own interests!

"So, what would you like to do?" I asked, holding my breath, wondering how far away from the baseball field he was about to take me.

"I want to hang out in the woods."

I thought about this. What would happen if I listened to Jack with my heart instead of my head? What were my expectations about anyway? After all, cooperation and teamwork can be learned just as well in the wild as on a ball field.

In that moment I packed up my expectations and let myself follow the heart of my child. I let go of the idea of putting Jack into what we, his parents, thought he should be doing and went back to what is at the foundation of the Life Map – helping Jack realize his potential to be the best that he can be.

Outside Influences
Influences can come from anywhere, from the messages that our own parents and teachers drummed into us to what we hear from the media, the movies, or around the office water cooler. There is nothing wrong with outside influences as long as we can separate what we believe from what we are told to believe. Other people's opinions and attitudes easily end up coloring our own. Being an objective observer and being aware of what you believe will help you determine your own mind-set.

Once you free yourself from your fears and insecurities, your specific expectations and dreams, and the expectations of others, and leave yourself open to the possibilities, you are in a much better position in your heart and mind to accept what comes your way and see the good in it.

REWIRING YOUR MIND

It is not surprising that how you see the world impacts your mind-set. Your perspective is based on your experiences, your unique history, your personality and character particularities, and the influence of others. However, how you see the world today does not have to be how you see the world tomorrow. Your mind-set can be changed. Here are some ways to do it.

Know your ingoing stance – Be aware of the biases, attitudes, philosophy, and perceptions that impact how you see the world. The more you are conscious of what is driving how you think, the more you can be in control of it.

Use an open approach – If you truly want to change the way that you think about something, start by being open and positive as you look at how you currently view the person or situation. You will never change a thing if you are negative all the way down the line.

Change your lens – Besides taking an open approach, change the way that you view the situation. This can be anything from putting aside biases to giving someone the benefit of the doubt to start fresh.

Commit to changing your mind-set – You swear that you will start fresh, and in fact you do for the first few days or so. But it is so easy to fall back into old patterns. Little by little, you are back to your old tricks before you know it. To make sure this does not happen, write down key words describing the mind-set that you want to have on an index card and leave it on your desk or somewhere visible as a reminder of what you want to accomplish.

PUTTING WHAT YOU'VE LEARNED INTO ACTION

Now that you've gained an understanding of your self-set, heart-set, and mind-set and how they affect your relationship with your child, try the following exercise.

ARE YOU A CHAMELEON?

Write down something that your child does that upsets, annoys, or frustrates you.

_____

Think about a situation that went badly when your child was doing this thing. Write down three things that you could have done differently. Don't worry about what your child's response would have been to these specific actions. Just focus on your own behavior.

1. _____

2. _____

3. _____

The next time that your child does whatever it is that upsets, annoys, or frustrates you, try one of the three responses that you wrote down that you think might have the best outcome. Write down what happened and how you both felt afterward.

_____

_____

_____

If things turned out better, you probably changed your mind-set and/or heart-set. If things did not improve, try one of the other approaches the next time. Eventually, you will find a way of responding and interacting that makes the situation go better and that improves your attitude.

Collectively, your self-set, mind-set, and heart-set are what guides your thinking, and ultimately your behavior. If these three are behind who you are and what you do, they hold a lot more weight than just providing a bit of insight into who you are. Ultimately, they are the ones that will determine what you stand for. And that is what constitutes the most important part of your being – your core values. Now let's see what role the core values play in your part of unfolding your child's tent.

THE BOTTOM LINE

- While you can't fundamentally change who you are, you can try to understand yourself better. Understanding your self-set will allow you to navigate your heart and mind to compensate for what you'd like to change but have a hard time doing.

- How you feel about your child often affects how you treat him. Recognizing your feelings is the first step toward changing your heart-set. Taking charge of your feelings and concentrating on the positive will help move your negative feelings to a better place.

- Your attitudes and perceptions affect how you see your child. The more that you can let go of your expectations and judgmental opinions, be open to new paths, and embrace change, the better off you will be.

- To change anything – the self-set, heart-set, or your mind-set – means starting at the bottom, with introspection.

CHAPTER 2

THE BULL'S EYE

Getting in Touch with Your Core Values

Your core values are at the very foundation of who you are. They are the set of ethics, morals, standards, principles, or rules that govern how you conduct yourself, treat others, and, in general, relate to the world. Decisions, behaviors, and attitudes come from them. They are what is underneath your heart-set and your mind-set.

Each of us comes into the world with a certain temperament that predisposes us to see the world in a certain way. Add to that mix the training, teaching, and influence of our parents, teachers, and others in our community, and you have the foundation of a person's core values.

Because our core values guide our actions and are reflected in our behaviors, it is important to be conscious of them. Being aware of who we are at our core allows us to step back and say, "Do I like how I act and what I am guided by?," and gives us the opportunity to make changes. Without self-awareness, we may, and often do, act in ways that are not consistent with what we truly believe but perhaps only satisfy some immediate need. Whether we are aware of it or not, every one of us is guided by a set of core values.

As you did with your heart-set and mind-set, reflecting on what is at the core of how you feel, how you think, and how you behave moves you from a reactive to a proactive position. Intention can replace impulse and lead you to a more deliberate life that reflects what you believe in. Taking a little time to think about what core principles or standards are important to you and how you want them reflected in your life is particularly important when you have extraordinary challenges in your life. Here's why.

Because our child's disability may impact his ability to follow social and behavioral norms, he may behave in ways that upset, frustrate, embarrass, and anger us. However hard we work on heart-set and mind-set, sometimes trying to stay in control and behave as we want pushes us beyond what we are capable of. And that's when having core values to fall back on – or to lead us forward – is invaluable.

When you can't get the feelings and the attitudes lined up with where you want them to be, you can go a layer deeper to those values or principles that can take you past what you are feeling and thinking to what you believe is the "right" thing for you to do. That is, your core values can get you over your reactive self by reminding you what your perspective *ought* to be and can help you realign your actions with your beliefs. Operating out of this deeper core can save you from sliding down many a slippery slope, as illustrated in the following holiday story.

One of our family's holiday traditions is to join my sister and her family and my mother for a day in New York City in early December. This is a challenge for Jack, but a tradition that I believe is important for our family and for him. One year Jack was so distracted that my husband had to bail out with him and take the train home halfway through a show. Another year, Jack was so wound up by the end of the day that my sister, an occupational therapist, ended up throwing pillows on him to give him the sensory input that she thought his body was asking for. Now, that was a long ride home.

The year when Jack was ten, the chosen show was "A Christmas Carol" at Madison Square Garden. I knew that the only way Jack would be able to stay tuned at such an overwhelming place and event was if he was practically on stage. I bought tickets almost as soon as they went on sale and was able to get up close, in the second row.[16]

---

[16] Making it a point, ahead of time, to think about the setting and what modifications or particularities would increase the chances of success for your child is well worth the effort.

I had decided to have everyone meet for lunch before the show; this would give us a chance to visit, and I felt it was a safer bet for in-control behavior from the kids than having them sit still in a restaurant after a two-hour show.

After a successful lunch, we headed to the show, setting out for the ten blocks between the restaurant and the theater. Keeping a group together is no easy feat under normal circumstances; keeping them together during the holiday season in New York City is a major accomplishment. How was I going to keep Jack, who always walked – no, ran – to the beat of his own drum, with the group?

We all began walking, skirting this way and that around the vendors, tourists, and New Yorkers all trying to get where they were going and out of the cold as quickly as possible. The smell of roasted nuts and salted pretzels – both trademarks of the city – soon greeted us. Jack stopped in front of a vendor and asked me if he could buy roasted peanuts. I could see the rest of my family, John included, rousing with negative responses.

"We just ate!" my three-square-meals-a-day mother immediately reacted.

I asked myself the question that frequently comes to mind: "What's the big deal if I say yes?" The truth of the matter was that Jack had been so excited to see his cousins that he had barely taken a bite of pizza at lunch.

"Sure," I said, handing him a ten-dollar bill. Never one to miss an opportunity for social training, I added, "but it's not polite to eat in front of others without offering them some too."

Jack had begun to see the benefits of playing the benevolent role, so he asked the vendor for four bags – one each for his sister, two cousins, and himself.

"That will be $10.25," the peanut man said, extending his hand to complete the sale.

Now it would have been simple to give Jack the extra $.25. But I saw he was handling the transaction and experience quite well, so I thought I'd raise the bar one more notch. "Gee, Jack, I'm sorry, but that's all we're going to spend on peanuts," I replied when asked for the extra money.

"But what will I do?" he asked, not seeing a mathematical solution to four children and three bags.

"How about sharing?" I suggested, knowing full well that the other children had grandly eaten their pizza and would not be wanting a full bag of nuts.

By this time, my rather disgusted family had headed off down the street, but I had the tickets so I knew they wouldn't go too far. I decided to take a little time to enjoy Jack and our time together. Walking along and holding hands, Jack and I looked this way and that, talking about what we saw around us. Sure enough, we caught up with the family four blocks later, played pass the nuts around, and had plenty of time to spare. No harm done. And Jack got an opportunity to be a momentary hero, thanks to the street vendor.

A year ago, I might have felt embarrassed (that would be my heart-set kicking in) that Jack wouldn't accept his grandmother's admonition that we had just eaten and started thinking, "Why can't my kid just do what we say?" (that would be my mind-set). When it comes to Jack, however, one of my core principles is "Seek first to understand." Rather than judge and put him into my own set of expectations, I stepped back and looked at Jack. He was overexcited and hungry because he hadn't eaten his lunch, so why not? The peanuts were right on the way. Another one of my general guiding principles is "Treat others kindly," so letting Jack buy the peanuts would be an opportunity for him to do this. It was a great opportunity for teaching.

Stepping back and looking at what really mattered (i.e., what is at my core) allowed me to handle the situation in a way that was successful for everyone. Jack's hunger was satisfied, the cousins got an unexpected treat, and Jack had the opportunity to work on his ability to share.

What's at Your Core?

A fifteen-year-old decides to drop piano lessons after ten years of hard study. She says that she isn't "into it" any more. Her parents are furious. "After all the money and running around we've done with you," her mother comments, "this is the thanks that we get?"

It is easy to look at what your child is (or isn't) doing or what he is (or isn't) accomplishing and get hooked into a way of being that has a particular image or standard of success or any number of things at its core. In the case of the dropped piano lessons, the mother was more wrapped up in the image of having a child with special achievements and how that reflected upon her than on what the girl wanted for herself.

Complete the following exercise to see what is driving your behaviors and thinking.

What's at Your Core

Think about how you spend your free time and work time and what drives your behaviors and thinking. Look at the following and rate the importance of each in your life by putting 1 next to the most important, 2 next to the second most important, and so on. If there are things that are not listed that are critical in your life, add them on the blank lines. This exercise is designed to open up your self-awareness.

_____ Family	_____ Self	_____
_____ Pleasure	_____ Possessions	_____
_____ Work	_____ Money	_____
_____ Principles	_____ Success	

There are many different core values that we can end up with. Take a minute to think about what yours are. Do they reflect the guideposts for your heart and mind?

What Are Your Core Values?

Circle all of the values below that you believe you exhibit.

Compassion	Loyalty	Kindness
Sensitivity	Tolerance	Strong-mindedness
Courage	Understanding	Bravery
Honesty	Patience	Equality
Trustworthiness	Humor	Empathy
Integrity	Sincerity	

How They All Connect – Heart, Mind, Self, and Core Values

Did you ever meet someone who bubbles forth enthusiasm and positive energy? You leave her and you are refreshed and energized. What is it about that person that makes you want to have some of what she's got? It is her upbeat attitude, joyful perspective, and radiant disposition.

Heart-set, mind-set, self-set, and core values are all connected. How you feel influences your attitude and thinking. (Your heart-set is impacting your mind-set.) How you see and think about someone influences how you feel about him. (Your mind-set influences your heart-set.) And how you feel about him affects your view of him. (Back to your heart-set influencing your mind-set.) Your heart-set and mind-set keep reinforcing one another, and they are both colored by the lens through which you see the world – your self-set.

But your core values, if they are truly the unbending, unchanging truths that you have chosen to live by, do not have this two-way relationship. What you feel and what you think at any particular moment should not have the power to change what you *believe*. What you believe should be reflected in everything that you feel, think, say, and do.

How you approach the world and how you interact with and relate to others is completely in your control. You may not think so at first, but look carefully. Is there anyone who has the power to tell you who you should be or how you should act? No. In the end, it is all up to you.

When you become aware of your feelings, attitudes, perceptions, and disposition, you are in a position to do something about them. Every person can change any or all of these things. But in order to do so, you have to be open and willing to change.

Reflections

Before we move on, take some time by yourself to think deeply about who you are and who you want to be. Do this over several days or weeks – sit with your initial ideas and see if they are truly authentic. When you are satisfied with them, fill in the sentences on the following page.

WHO AM I AND WHAT I WANT TO BE

Core Values

My core values are:

_____

_____

_____

I want my core values to be:

_____

_____

_____

Self-Set

If I had to tell a stranger about myself, here is what I would say:

_____

_____

_____

Heart-Set

When I think about my child, these "feeling" words come to mind:

_____

_____

_____

Mind-Set

When I think about my child, my overall attitude is:

_____

_____

If Life Mapping is more or less a roadmap, then core values are the rules of the road. Can you imagine driving in a foreign country or even another state and not being clear about the road rules? Can I take a right on red or not? Is passing allowed only on the left? Is the posted speed limit the true limit, or is it my father's rule of thumb that you can go eight miles above before you tick the police officer off?

You are a much more effective and safe driver when you know the road rules. Similarly, you have a much greater chance of acting in a way that is consistent with what you believe if you know what you believe in. That said, each of us probably does not need to look very far to think of someone who says she believes in one thing, but acts in a different way. It is always easier to think about being good, or kind or whatever virtue you hold dear, than to act it. And that little dilemma takes us right to the next chapter – actions speak louder than words.

THE BOTTOM LINE

- Your core values are the set of ethics, morals, standards, principles, or rules that govern how you conduct yourself, treat others, and relate to the world.

- Your core values should underlie all important decisions in your life.

- Your heart-set, mind-set, self-set, and core values are interconnected. How you feel influences your attitude and thinking, and vice versa. And what you believe in affects your attitude and your feelings.

CHAPTER 3

You Are Who You Act

Actions Speak Louder Than Words

Living by what you believe in and getting your heart and mind in a healthy place is no small feat. You might think that with all the work you've just done you are ready to go on cruise control. Not quite. We still need to talk about your behaviors and actions.

You can have the best core values in the world, but if you don't live by them, they are hollow. Similarly, how you feel and think and how you act is your responsibility. You can behave more like you want to by changing your heart-set or your mind-set, and by gaining more self-control. To do so, you must begin with conscious actions and try to make them regular habits. Remember when you were learning how to drive a car? In the first few days, you were very precarious and tried to do each thing in precisely the correct way, from moving the stick shift to parallel parking. It felt as if the world's eyes were on you when you started to drive. And now look at you: talking on your cell phone, forefinger and thumb doing the two-step on the steering wheel, and music blaring. How to drive is engrained in you and has become automatic. This is how habits are – automatic.

When your core values, heart-set, mind-set, and self-set are lined up and reflected in correct actions, you are living a "process-oriented life."[17] When you are process-driven, you are more concerned with the journey than with the endpoint. The endpoint is important as a reference, but you recognize that you will change as a result of your journey, and that, more than reaching the goal, is the most important thing.

Being centered means that you are grounded in your approach. Even if things happen that are unexpected and do not go your way, they do not unsettle you. Because you are principle-centered, you are grounded in truths that do not change based on time, person, place, or thing. Because you orient your heart-set to joy and your mind-set is positive, you remain hopeful.

Once you have your mind, heart, and soul oriented in a true direction, and your behaviors are no longer impulsive but process-oriented, you will see yourself change. And when you change, the nature of your relationship with others changes, even if they do nothing at all. And that is the beginning of successful relationship building.

GOOD ACTIONS ARE LIKE PUTTING MONEY IN THE BANK

Every time we have an encounter with someone, it is either an investment or a withdrawal. If we have an exchange where the other person feels good and we do too, it is an affirming, building experience. Like making a deposit in an account, we are depositing goodwill in the relationship. Conversely, when there is an exchange or interaction that is not so good, something is taken away from the relationship. It is left with less in it than before. The feelings, the mind-set, and the values that I say I have are all deposits in my relationship with my son.

LINING UP WHAT YOU SAY WITH WHAT YOU DO

Part of getting your inside self in sync with your outside self (what others see) involves being conscious of the dynamics of the "relationship account." But just being conscious of it is not enough. You have to make some changes and take some action.

One way of doing this is to acquire some better habits. Take a minute and complete the exercise on the following page to begin to get a better understanding of this.

---

[17]   The concept of process-oriented living is taken from Robin Kencel and Susan Eberhardt, *I Only Have a Minute So This Better Be Good* (Greenwich, CT: Publication pending).

TAKING A CLOSER LOOK AT YOUR ACTIONS

1. Write down three behaviors or ways that you interact with your child that usually leads to positive outcomes:

   1. _____

   2. _____

   3. _____

2. Write down three behaviors or ways that you interact with your child that usually leads to negative outcomes:

   1. _____

   2. _____

   3. _____

Once you recognize the behaviors that need adjusting, it is time to figure out a way to change them and then to transform these changed behaviors into habits.

GOOD HABITS ARE NOT HARD TO COME BY

In making the changes that you have decided to make, it might help to think of some sound bites that can spur you on. Sound bites, for our purposes, may be thought of as catchy little phrases or well-worn adages that are easy to remember. Whenever I get in a negative run of interactions with my children, I put myself on a little behavior chart. I jot down the behaviors that I want to change and then attach little rewards for changing them; like treating myself to a new book when I have been patient with the children for an entire week. After that, I develop a sound bite to help me remember what it is that I am doing – something that captures what I want to be. Here is a sample of some sound bites that have been helpful to me:

- Seek first to understand.

- Acceptance, not expectation.

- It's *not* all about me.

- It's all in the approach.

What you adopt for your sound bites should reflect your priorities.

The Five R's

If you want to change yourself – your inside self – think about it in terms of the five R's:

1. *Reflect* – Look at how you act, how you spend your time, what you think about, how you define success (for yourself, your children, and your family), and determine what has been your "engine."

2. *Revamp* – Think through what you want your core values to be and write them down some place where you will be reminded of what they are.

3. *Respond* – Every action is an investment or a withdrawal. Act in a way that is consistent with what your beliefs (values) are.

4. *Relax* – This does not have to be an intense, big-deal thing. No one is perfect, and you are not expected to set that up as a goal. Enjoy the process along the way.

5. *Rejoice* – As your relationships improve, rejoice. The payoff of a better relationship is a big one. Recognize that.

You might be wondering why we are spending so much time on core values and how they are played out in real life in a book that is about helping and supporting a child in reaching his potential. It has to do with foundations. If we want to empower our children, we must act in ways that model what we hope to train in him. With all your self-knowledge you are in the driver's seat instead of being one of those reactive backseat drivers. In the end, the more self-aware you are, the more you can be in control of your actions, including how you interact with your child. Let's take a look at your relationship with your child right now.

- When you are operating with a clear heart-set and mind-set and are intentional in your actions, your actions will reflect your inside self, who you are and who you hope to be.

- A relationship is like a bank account, you have investments and withdrawals. To end up with a healthy account, be sure that you invest more (more positive interactions) than you take out (negative experiences).

- Remember the five "R's" – reflect, revamp, respond, relax, and rejoice.

CHAPTER 4

RAGAMUFFIN RELATING

Fostering a Satisfying Relationship with Your Child

*O*ne day, a student in the eleventh grade named Les went into one of the class-rooms at his school looking for a friend. Noticing Les, the teacher, Mr. Washington, asked him to go to the blackboard.

Les replied, "But, I'm not one of your students."

Mr. Washington said, "It doesn't matter. Go to the board anyhow." Les told the teacher that he couldn't do that. When Mr. Washington asked him why, Les told him it was because he had Down's Syndrome.[18]

At this point Mr. Washington walked over to him and said, "Don't you ever say that again. Someone's opinion of you does not have to become your reality."

It was a liberating moment for Les, and Mr. Washington ended up becoming his mentor. Over the years, while other teachers passed Les from class to class, Mr.

---

[18] Since that time, it's been determined that whatever hes had, if anything, was not Down's Syndrome.

Washington made more demands of him, made him accountable, and enabled him to believe in himself. He gave him a larger vision of himself.

Les Brown and his orchestra became one of the leading swing bands in the country. When asked what he attributes his fame to, Les never fails to mention Mr. Washington for giving him a sense of destiny.

Working from the inside-out[19] is a good way to approach life and your relationships. There is much about yourself that you can control – your approach, your attitude, and, to a certain extent, even your temperament. And you can certainly control your behaviors. What you cannot control is what the other person thinks or feels, or how she acts.

Your relationship with your child is not going to be picture-perfect. It may not be a conventional relationship, but it can still be fulfilling.

Do You Know How Important You Are?

Have you ever seen a child who has made a U-turn and is now heading in the right direction? You can't believe how far along he has come. You wonder how it happened. Was it an alternative therapy? A medication? A miracle? Luck? In qualitative research[20] I asked educators, "What do you think is the single biggest factor in a child who makes a big shift?" By "big shift" we mean not just steady progress, although we'd love that, but the knock-you-over, can't-believe-that's-the-same-kid kind of a change. The answer, almost unanimously, was having someone who believes in the child.

We have an enormous opportunity to make a significant difference in the child's life. This is true for parents, teachers, coaches, therapists, or anyone who regularly interacts with the child. Mr. Washington didn't just "happen" to connect with Les Brown. Mr. Washington operated from a personal philosophy that believed in the intrinsic worth and potential of all children. And he acted in a way that was consistent with his beliefs.

Developing the Relationship

"What does your child do that really upsets you?" That was the question I posed to parents in a lecture on how to manage children with ADHD more effective-

---

[19] Inside-out terminology is taken from Stephen Covey, *Seven Habits of Highly Effective People* (New York: Fireside Books, 1989).

[20] Fifteen one-on-one interviews conducted with educators at the elementary and middle-school levels.

ly. Someone in the back of the room said in a low whisper, "Everything." Nervous laughter followed. A mother then raised her hand and said, "I ask my child when she walks in the door from school how her day was, and she says, 'I don't want to talk about it.'" She went on, "After she doesn't want to talk about it, she eats something that she isn't supposed to. I ask her to change out of her school clothes and begin her homework, but she ignores both of my requests and just does her own thing."

In this situation, it seems that the mother is more interested in getting through her agenda and having the child fit her schedule than what is best for the child. This is not to say that the mother should let the child ignore her question, eat what she wants, and begin homework "whenever," but it does mean that the mother must look at what is going on from her daughter's perspective and capabilities. School was probably emotionally and physically draining. The last thing the child needs is to walk in the door only to be met with further demands in the first few minutes. She most likely needs some downtime to unwind and let the pressure of the day melt away. The mother would be far better off talking with her daughter about how much time might be good for taking an initial break, perhaps setting a timer and having the child begin homework and the after-school routine when the timer goes off.

Most children who are in fourth or fifth grade can participate in some way and need to start being part of setting their own time schedule and taking responsibility. When they were younger, they might have been given a visual schedule to follow along with auditory devices such as a timer. But as they get older, they need to begin learning how they are going to train themselves to manage their time and their responsibilities. This makes the child a partner in the process and empowers him.

Following are guideposts that can help you in taking the leaps to change your heart and your mind, and that will change your relationship with your child.

1. *Measure success in a new way.* Parents measure the success of their child – and often their own success – by what their child achieves. Who hasn't been around a father or mother who can't help but brag about their son's pitching ability, his grades, teams he was chosen for, and schools he got accepted to? As a society we place value on goals and achievements, and we look to our children to be part of this game, even when we don't mean to.

Your child will have his share of successes, but they will not necessarily be the typical successes for children of his age. That doesn't matter. It is important for you to view your child, his growth, and his progress against a success standard that is fair for him. If you want to have a real relationship with your child, you need to change your view on what it means for him to be successful. If you don't, you will nearly always be disappointed, which will affect your heart-set. If you are able to change your mind-set on how you measure success in your child, you will be on a journey that leads to celebrating the gains and developments throughout his life.

2. *Reframe your expectations of "rewards."* Ahhh, the rewards of parenting. All of us have expectations of what those rewards will be. To see our children's eyes light up when we enter a room; to be that "special person" in their life that they come to for advice and comfort; to hear their after-school tales and impart our great wisdom to them; to see them do well in school, be accepted to and attend an excellent college; marry and have children of their own … The list goes on and on.

Maybe for a child who lives in his own world, the greatest reward would be for him to reach out to you. Perhaps you have a child who is propelled by his own agenda, and your reward is the day that he follows one of your directions for the first time. For me, one of my greatest rewards was the day when Jack held my hand as we crossed the street and made our way to the speech therapist's office. Now that he is eleven, reward is seeing him bring home a play date from school.

You can enjoy great rewards in parenting your child, if you know where to look.

3. *Let the team raise the child; let the village raise you.* As we will discuss in the next section, your child will be supported by a team or many teams. That is a given. But what about you? Where do you go to refill the cup that will refresh you?

Having a circle of support – a few friends, a family member, and perhaps even a mental health professional – that you trust and feel free to share your honest feelings with is indispensable. You must have people whom you can lean on and let down your hair with. At every developmental stage in your child's life that is missed or gone through shakily, you will grieve and wish for what could be. The daily disappointments, combined with recurring setbacks and crises, require the listening, nonjudgmental ear of a good friend or other support person.

Do not try to be a hero by going it solo. There are people around you who are willing and wanting to be a support. Let them. The more you feel strong and rested, the more energy and stamina you will have to make the extra effort to reach your child.

4. *Meet the child where he is.* If you don't accept this, not only are you not going to change where the child is, you will have started off on the most negative foot imaginable. Meeting the child where he is will help you to develop a positive relationship with him.

5. *Accentuate the positive, eliminate the negative.* It has been said that children with special needs receive fifteen negative comments for every compliment. How does that stack up in your household? If you encourage your children along the way to identify their feelings and express them, you may find that they will let you know when your negative spin is too much for them. When that happens, it is time to ramp up the positive and take down the negative. Even if it is something as small as letting them know that you liked the way that they walked in the door or closed the refrigerator after they got a snack, do it. The more you tell your child that you liked what he did, the more he will want to do more of it – and the more you will get yourself in a positive frame of mind.

6. *Listen first.* How come we love to hear ourselves talk so much? Did you ever notice how people often talk instead of listen? I do it myself. My children begin to tell me something that happened in school and immediately I want to tell them what I think and how to fix it. I can't help myself. After all, I have been there.

When we listen to our children, we are telling them (without words) that we value what they are thinking and what they have to say. This can be incredibly empowering, especially to the child who feels that he is talked "at" all day long. Try a little listening and see if it doesn't make a difference in your relationship with him.

7. *Get rid of your own agenda.* Agendas are dangerously close to expectations, and we have seen what those can do to a child. When we focus too much on our own agenda, we can forget what is best for our child and get wrapped up in what is important only to ourselves. If you are honestly focused on working off your child's interests and accepting him where he is today, you will not have any hidden, or not-so-hidden, agendas going on at the same time.

8. *Separate the child from you.* The more you invest yourself, your time, and your resources in the life of your child, the easier it is for you to lose your focus and perspective. For your own peace of mind, and also for the mental health of your family, it is important that you keep up hobbies, interests, or whatever passions have typically given you pleasure and been part of who you are. The parent who says, "I used to work out regularly, but now, because of our 'situation,' I just don't have the time," is not only doing herself an injustice but is not helping her family either.

9. *Magnify the feeling of being loved.* Since many emotions and feelings in the typical world completely bypass your child on any given day, good or bad, you might want to think about the concept of "broadcasting" positive feedback in the beginning. John was the all-time king of this when Jack was little. "Hey, Jack, how much do I love you?" John would ask the minute he walked in the door from work. It didn't matter that Jack would ignore him for the first twenty minutes. At regular intervals, John would ask his question again, coming right up to where Jack was. If Jack didn't answer, John would answer for him. And he did this until his son gave him the answer he was waiting for. That was in the tough years, of which there were several. As Jack became more "versed" in social skills and began to learn what feelings and connecting were about, something finally gave way inside of him. The connections began happening. The other day when I was helping him organize his friends to enter a frisbee tournament, Jack turned to me and said, "You were the best today. I could never have gotten all that organizing done without you." That sounds pretty close to a feelings compliment to me. But we didn't just get there suddenly one day. It took years of building the emotional scaffolding – big and tall and very visible for him to see.

One more point on this. We have tried to be very careful about what Jack has watched on television. Using books and videos to provide your child with examples of healthy emotional relating, appropriate behaviors, certain values or attributes, or whatever it is you are trying to emphasize at the time can be very powerful.

MAYBE IT'S JUST A DIFFERENT LANGUAGE

Think of your child in this way: What if all babies in the world were supposed to be born knowing how to speak and understand our language and most of them actually did but you were one of the families that got a baby who spoke a different language? At first, you tried to force him to speak English, but he refused to speak at all. So you moved to the reward system. But that was exhausting and, besides, after a little while he was on to your game. At your wits' end one day, you wondered what would happen if you tried to learn a little of your baby's language. You did, and you saw the beauty in it. In fact, the world looked different to you when spoken in a different language. And most interesting of all, as your baby saw you making the effort to learn his language, he decided to explore yours. You didn't say a word. You didn't correct him. You only applauded the effort. Soon, you were building bridges instead of fences.[21]

Meet your child where he is, focusing on the positive and using it to build a bridge to help him reach you and others.

THINK LOW AND SLOW

As a rule of thumb, think about meeting the child "low" and "slow." When you meet a child low, you are meeting him at or below his eye level. A child who is being talked to from above is instantly intimidated. Don't relate from an imposing level. Bend down, sit, or do what it takes to get eyeball to eyeball with the child.

Get low in your voice as well. By bringing down your volume and your pitch, you also bring down the intensity of the interaction. Practice a soft tone of voice. Your child might be extra sensitive to sound or tone.

Finally, move slowly and calmly. A child whose motor is overcharged, experiences some level of anxiety, or in some way has difficulty finding his own center, will respond better and be helped by having someone who is modeling self-control, moving deliberately and carefully. The child plays off of the energy and dynamics set by those around him; the more you are mindful of the modeling you are providing here, the more you will serve the needs of the child.

HELP YOUR CHILD UNDERSTAND HIMSELF

Parents often ask me if they should let their child know what he "has." My answer is a resounding "Yes!" However, this information must be shared at the right time and in the right way. The right time is when you feel that your child is cognitively and emotionally ready. He is ready when he begins to exhibit a willingness and an ability to take at least some responsibility for his behaviors. There is no sense in discussing with him why self-control is important if he has no concept of what self-control is, for example.

---

[21] James Dobson, *Bringing up Boys: Practical Advice and Encouragement for Those Shaping the Next Generation of Men* (Carol Stream, IL: Tyndale House Publishing, 2001).

The first conversation I had with Jack about his disorder occurred when he was nine years old. He had just come home from day camp and was riding his bike up and down the driveway. The day camp he was attending was for children with ADHD, developmental delays, and related disorders. Although I had screened the camp and had thought the level of disability of the other children matched Jack's level of functioning, it turned out that socially and emotionally most of the children were more severe than I had anticipated. Jack was picking up some pretty bad language and behaviors.

I asked Jack to put his bike away and go in the house to wash up while I ran to town to pick up something that I needed for dinner. But he wasn't interested in stopping his biking right then and there. To let me know his displeasure, he sat down a few feet in front of my car.

"Jack! What are you doing?" I said, getting out of the car and standing over him.

"This is what the kids at camp would do," he said, looking up

"But those kids have severe special needs," I said, not thinking about what I was saying.

Jack looked at me incredulously, "So why am I there?"

This was the opportunity I had been waiting for. Jack had made some strong behavioral gains in the past school year. I felt he was ready to hear the basic components of his disorder. My goal was to include him as a partner in the process of overcoming or working around his issues.

In a calm, matter-of-fact voice, I explained Jack's uniqueness to him: "You know how wonderfully well you work alone. You do a great job whenever you have a project you do by yourself. But in life, it will be important for you to be able to work with others on projects, too. You were made in such a way that working in a group doesn't come easily for you. And that's what we'll be working on. That's why you are at The Viceroy Camp – you are learning how to play and work with other kids."

That was all I needed to say that day. The seed had been sown, and at appropriate times, when Jack was starting to follow only his own agenda, I gently pointed out what he was doing and described how it might seem to others. Of course,

I only suggested this at times when I felt fairly confident that he had the capacity to overcome a given behavior.

Be careful about doing this though. You do not want your child to begin to feel labeled or to feel put down in any way. I would not suggest this tact if you are in any way upset or angry with him because it could come off as insulting and demeaning. I would only use this strategy when there is a specific behavior that you feel your child could extinguish (and would be motivated to) if he realized what he was doing and how it affected others.

You Bet It's Worth It

It's up to you to build the scaffolding to reach your child. This is not for the fainthearted. Or for those just trying to get by. Or for those who aren't interested in challenges. Ragamuffin relating – meeting the child however you can to engage with him and elicit a response of some sort – is a fine way to start. But your ultimate goal is to move him from a ragamuffin, come-as-you-are sort of stage to an interaction that is on a more equal footing. This can happen if you, with the help of others, take the time to build the scaffolding that will support the bridge.

You might think of your relating to your child like this. In the early years when his barriers are high and his abilities are at their lowest, it is up to you and others who work with him to build whatever support is needed to reach where he is, emotionally and socially. You can begin to work with him to build a footbridge to the typical world. Since he will be part of this building process, you will be able to take some cues from him, observing what he responds well to, seeing what works and what doesn't. As he makes the connections, overcomes things that stand in his way, and figures out how to negotiate the challenges, you can slowly begin removing the scaffolding, bit by bit.

By developing a Life Map for your child, you will have a blueprint for just what to build and when to build it. As your child reaches new developmental heights, he will be able to learn strategies to help him cope and even successfully negotiate in a social world that is otherwise mostly foreign to him. Eventually, he will figure out an architecture for his life that is part bridges, part detours, and part long, hard hauls. The more that you serve as a positive support, the more he will have the structure he needs to adapt to the world.

The Players – One Person at a Time

I hope you now have a greater sense of who you are and why you act as you do. Add to that a greater understanding of your child, and you have the ingredients for better interactions and, hopefully, better relationships – not just between you and your child, but with anybody. I come from a family of four children, and I was always struck by how exponentially noisy and complicated dinnertime would become, depending upon the number of children at the table. Of course, this makes sense once you think about it mathematically. One child at the table with two adults means that four different interactions can occur. That is, four different opportunities for getting along – or not. Add just one more child to the table and there are now eight different interactions and double the number of opportunities for joy or upset. The more people that are added to a relationship, the more complicated things can become. Much of life is more than one-on-one relationships. Working as part of a group brings with it a whole new level of complexity.

The teams that support your child can be a critical component of his progress. Having mastered understanding yourself and your child is a great start, but if you think that's all there is to helping him reach his potential, you are ignoring a powerful piece that can help get him there – the team. Like everything in life, there are good teams and not-so-good teams. Now, with a better sense of who you are and what you might want to change or think about to become an even better you, let's look at you in a different light – as a member of one of the most important teams that you will ever be on – the one that supports your child.

- You can't control anyone's actions outside your own, but you can control your approach, your attitude, and your behaviors. How your relationship with your child develops is in your hands as much as it is in his, if not more.

- It may not be *exactly* the relationship that you had in mind, but if you are flexible and more focused on the process than on a specific way that things "ought to be," you can have a successful relationship with your child.

- Meeting the child where he is, is just the first step on a journey toward a path where you can eventually walk together, if you are willing to take the time to build some bridges along the way.

PART III

THE PROCESS

SECTION 1

A TEAM APPROACH
An Introduction to Teams

An Introduction to Teams

Not only did most of us receive little if any training on parenting, we are even less prepared for how to parent a child who is one-of-a-kind. When we finally figured out that we had one of these children, most of us went into immersion mode, learning everything that we could get our hands on. And what many of us learned is that much of what our children need to grow and manage requires training that we do not have. Luckily for us, specialized therapists, teachers, and doctors are often at our fingertips to provide the services that our children need.

The reality of a team is that it can bring together the resources and skills that one individual rarely possesses. The better a team functions, the better the outcomes will be. If the team is organized properly and the members have the skills necessary to effectively do their job, the work can be done. If there is a process in place that encourages and supports the team, the delivery of services to your child will be one of continual improvement. And, if the team's underlying norms and values are carefully conceived, the team will be focused on the right things, and the right things will be achieved.

This book assumes that you already know the basics of how a team, particularly a school-based team, operates. The purpose of talking about process and teams is to explore how you can make an impact and influence the teams that are supporting your child, making contributions that only parents can make. We will do this largely in the context of what we've already examined in you and in your relationship with your child through looking at the heart-set and mind-set of the team.

Because a team is made up of individuals, it creates a heart-set and mind-set of its own, whether the team members recognize it or not. And just as for an individual, the more the team's heart-set and mind-set are in the right place, the greater the chances for the most powerful work to be accomplished.

CHAPTER 1

Boot Camp Basics

You Are Part of a Bigger Picture

Who Makes up the Team?

Who makes up the team or teams that support your child will vary over the course of your child's life as his needs and functioning change. Anyone who is a regular part of your child's life can, and should, be thought of as a part of the team. The broader you envision the team, the more opportunities you will find for people to support and carry out the goals and strategies that have been established for your child.

For instance, if you think of the school-based team as only the classroom teacher and special services providers (such as therapists), you are missing out on the contributions that everyone from the art teacher to the lunchroom lady can – and most certainly do – make. Outside of school, the team should be thought of as including coaches, church school teachers, regular babysitters, and anyone in your extended family who has regular contact with your child.

In fact, anyone who satisfies the following criteria might be thought of as a part of the team:

- Is committed to the goals and strategies that have been articulated for your child

- Has regular contact with your child

- Has a positive impact on your child and advances the plan

You can think of the team supporting your child in two ways. One is the big team, which is made up of all the people who work with your child on a regular basis. This includes, but is not limited to:

- Your child

- Psychiatrist, psychopharmacologist, or other physician who prescribes medication

- Psychologist

- Speech and language, occupational, physical, vision therapists

- Social worker

- Teachers – inclusion, special education, "specials" (art, gym, music)

- Outside coaches and teachers (religious education, sports, etc.)

- Babysitters

- Family (grandparents, aunts and uncles, other family members who are a regular part of the child's life)

- Mentor, Big Brother/Big Sister

- Your child's friends and peers

The other team, which is the team that takes on greater importance as your child begins school, is a subset of this larger team. It is the school-based team. Based on legislation, the special education department at the board of education, or the folks in charge of special education at the school, decides who will be the core members of your child's school-based team. Who is on the team ultimately depends upon your child's needs.

Here we will focus on the school-based team. There are several reasons for this. First, although you can choose to end your relationship with a health care provider who is not working out, for example, you do not have the same flexibility with your school-based team. Who you get on your team is usually there to stay, so it is best to figure out how to make the situation work.

Second, the school is the place where most of the work with your child is done. Generally speaking, between the ages of three and eighteen, your child will be spending a significant and important period of time in a school-based setting.

SOME GENERAL RULES

The day-to-day life of a team consists of three things: the plan, the process, and the relationships of team members – with each other and with the child. Beyond trying to put into place the kind of self-reflection and actions discussed in the section on understanding yourself, certain basic attributes greatly enhance team functioning and the effectiveness of meetings, if everyone on the team practices them. This list is not meant to be exhaustive, but a starting point for you to begin looking at how your own behaviors might impact the team.

- *Leave the baggage home.* We *do not*, repeat *do not*, want to bring our emotional baggage to the team meeting. This message is particularly for parents. It helps for school staff to be aware that this is a tall order for parents to help them understand some of parents' behaviors.

Taking a little time before you get to a meeting to think through what it is you want to tell the team, what work has to get done in the meeting, and how much time the team has available will help you prioritize how long you can spend talking about your fears, worries, disappointments, and concerns related to your child.

- *Don't talk just to hear yourself talk.* Think through what main ideas you would like to get across and try to state them as succinctly as possible.

Teenagers are said to hear no more than the first seven words that adults say before they tune out; the average person probably doesn't hear much more.

- *Be solution-oriented.* If you bring up a problem, try to have some ideas for a solution ready at the same time. People who point out problems with no attempt to fix them may end up getting stuck in negative-negative land, a place where you do not want to be.

THE TEAM-PLAYER ROLES OF PARENTS

Contrary to what some believe, you are not a guest, a visitor, the boss, or the outside judge of the team. As a parent, you are part of the team and have a real role to play and responsibilities to meet. Although your role is often not as well laid out as the roles of the rest of the team members, whose roles and responsibilities are specified in their job descriptions and by the principal or leader in charge of the school's special needs program, parents nevertheless have specific roles and responsibilities on the team. In addition to the responsibilities that any general team member has, parents fulfill other key functions. Further, if you have skills that allow you to take on more of a leadership role within the team, and you can do it while maintaining an objective and fair perspective, by all means offer to do so.

Your involvement as the parent member of the team may change a bit each year, depending upon the type of year that your child is having. A tough year will call for more involvement; a good year will call for less. Although you may have a sense of when you need to be more or less involved, your role and responsibilities on the team from year to year may not be as clear to you. For example, if the team that will be supporting your child this year is new to you or different from the one that developed the IEP, you might want to sit down with all of them, or at least a few key members, to clarify their expectations of your role and responsibilities.

KEY RESPONSIBILITIES

Parents should have the same sense of accountability and role clarity as the rest of the team members. The worst thing a parent can do is to be part of a team, take no responsibility, and point out all the things that are not what they should be (at least in the parent's eyes). Being the passive observer, the angry force, or the negative naysayer does nothing to support the team, nor does it ingratiate you to the team. At a minimum, a parent has three responsibilities:

1. To be the source and coordinator of information

2. To establish the communication link between home and school

3. To support the school-based plan at home

If you aren't comfortable with these responsibilities, make it your commitment to your child to get the skills training necessary for you to uphold these responsibilities – and uphold them well.

Be the Source and Coordinator of Information
You have more information and more sources of important information about your child than anyone else. You need to share this information in a concise, clear way with the school team. A short memo that consolidates observations from your perspective, and perhaps from others outside the school who are working with your child, is extremely useful.[22]

For example, giving the school-based team a snapshot of what your child did during the summer with the objective of highlighting major issues and achievements, and perhaps reviewing the IEP to see if any issues need to be immediately addressed, can save time and guesswork in the first few weeks, when team members are getting to know your child along with eighteen or so other students.

I like to prepare quarterly memos for the school-based and outside teams that give them an overview of my child's progress. To that end, I ask team members to briefly write down or tell me the key goals that they are working on, gains that have been made, issues that have cropped up, and any concerns they have. This allows me to coordinate the information for the team to see. You may want to provide phone numbers or e-mail addresses in the memo so that team members can contact each other if they want to. If you do not have the skills necessary to prepare the memo, suggest the idea to the team and work with them to identify the best person to take on this job.

Establish the Communication Link
How much you need to be in communication with your child's teacher and other members of the team depends on the number and the severity of the issues and concerns you are dealing with. Every child will run into bumps. Don't wait for

---

[22] If you need help creating this sort of written communication, see the sample letters in the appendix of *One Small Starfish* (Arlington, TX: Future Horizons, 2003), pp. 290-294.

the issue to find its way to you. Ask your child's teacher what communication mode she prefers and then use it prudently. I have been able to head off bad ideas and get homework heads-ups by e-mailing Jack's teacher early in the morning. She checks her messages before the school day begins, and we are in sync before Jack's head pops through her classroom door.

Halfway through Jack's fifth-grade year, I heard of a well-respected social skills group being run by two social workers. With middle school just around the corner, I thought this class might be one last good and targeted run at social skills – something that Jack was less and less inclined to work on. It was a small-group format where the boys watched a movie segment and used that to work on specific issues that parents had identified as needing to be worked on. Jack was skeptical, but I gave him no choice – he at least had to try the class.

The focus of the first class was called "Getting the Big Picture and Letting the Details Go." The main idea was to train the boys to stick with the main issue of what was going on with them socially (i.e., to learn to increase their social awareness) and not get distracted with things that were unimportant or incidental. The next day, I e-mailed everyone on the school team, sharing the main points of the social skills class and asking them to use the phrase, "Now what's the big picture here?," to reinforce the concept with Jack during the week. Jack came home in an outrage.

"Did you tell any of my teachers that I am going to a social skills class?" he demanded as he walked in the door. I admitted that I had. "Well, tell them not to talk to me about 'the big picture.' I get the point, and it makes me sound like an idiot when they say that to me in front of the other kids."

There are several issues at stake here. As your child grows older and becomes more aware of his differences, he will likely have opinions or feelings about the interventions that have been put into place for him. When you think he is ready, it is important that your child feels that he is part of the team and has an opportunity to voice his opinion.

Should I have let Jack decide if he should participate in the social skills class? A few things should be taken into consideration in answering this question. First, the old story about leading a horse to water seems to fit. I knew that Jack had the capacity to not only get nothing from the class if he chose to, but also to disrupt the class. But letting him make the decision with the reason that "I don't need it, I don't have social issues" was not only incorrect, it meant losing an opportunity that in the long run might greatly benefit him. As a parent, I see my role as changing from a manager to a consultant – to the extent that I am able to share the decision-making process with Jack. But I can only do this if he has learned effective problem-solving skills and is able to reasonably and objectively analyze situations. This is a lot to expect from an eleven-year-old.

In this situation, I did not feel Jack had the understanding and maturity to decide if he should take the class, but I did know he could shut down and gain nothing from it if he went in with a negative mind-set. So I asked Jack if he thought he could make this compromise: He would attend one class and see how it went. If he hated the class and could give me two reasons why he shouldn't have to take it, we would revisit the decision. He went to the class. He gave me two reasons. They sounded somewhat reasonable but more important, I knew he wasn't open to learning at this point in time. I agreed that he could pass on the class but told him the specific social skills that the class was working on and said that I would be looking at these in the next few months. If I gave him repeated examples of his behavior that showed he could have benefited from the class, he would have to attend the next session.

Once the decision was made, I cycled back to the teachers to let them know what social skills I would be monitoring and asked them to do the same and what we had decided about the class. The decision to keep all the teachers in the loop and part of the support for the social skills class was a valid one. The fact that Jack was aware of what we were doing speaks to his improved self-awareness and ability to take on more responsibility for making changes himself.

Support the School-Based Plan at Home

Our job as parents is to teach our children good life habits. The job of the school is to teach in a way that children can learn. Letting your child eat what he wants, do his homework "whenever," go to bed when he feels like it, and spend his free time however he pleases is not teaching or modeling anything positive. Teaching good life habits to children who naturally have a hard time with the foundation of good habits – structure, time management, and organization – is necessary if you want them to be able to manage themselves later on in life.

If your child is working on specific behavior goals in school, it is important also to work on the goals at home. Doing this from day one makes good sense. Sit down with your child's teacher and any other key members of the school-based team the week before school, or the first week of school, to review how the behavioral, emotional, and social aspects of your child's plan will be handled so all of you are operating and responding in the same way. When the same thing is being done at home and at school, the volume control is doubled and your child can hear the messages more strongly in terms of understanding expectations and learning new skills.

Consistency at home and at school is what Life Mapping is all about. Although school may not have the broader goals that you are focusing on, there will be considerable overlap in the emotional and social areas. Whatever the top priorities are in school should be the same at home. If "learning to share" is a biggie at school, you'd better be working on it at home as well.

SUPPORT THE TEAM

Your presence on the team will impact the team either positively or negatively. If you want to be as effective as possible, you can do so by:

• Believing in and nurturing the talents of the other team members

• Encouraging and supporting team members to do their best work

• Demonstrating appreciation for the work of the team members

Who among us can't figure out how to believe in, nurture, encourage, support, and show appreciation to others? On the simplest level, parents can take on this aspect of being a leader. As mentioned, if parents are comfortable with other aspects of leadership, they can approach the team about taking those on as well. Depending on the team's dynamics, the comfort level of individual team members, and the strengths of the other team members, parents may become the coordinator and dissemination center for team information, or perhaps the facilitator or the scribe in meetings.

- Once the child enters school, the school-based team is usually the centerpoint of any team supporting the child. Use formal and informal channels of communication to keep team members informed and in contact with each other. Since the team does not formally meet often, it is important that team members find ways to stay in contact and share information on a regular basis.

- Specific roles and responsibilities of team members keep the team functioning effectively. It is good to articulate early in the life of the team what the team roles are and who will play them. The first step toward creating a successful team is having a team that is well designed and well run.

- Parents are well positioned to be the coordinators of information and supporters for the team. You have the advantage of having the best access to the child's outside therapists and other providers and can continue working on goals beyond the school day. Parents can also take on a leadership role on the team if they have the capabilities and feel comfortable doing so. Learning the tools necessary to play your role will be a major boost to the entire team and empower you as well.

CHAPTER 2

HEART-SET AND MIND-SET OF THE TEAM

What's Good for One Is Good for All

Our personal goals determine what we do and, to some extent, how we act. We saw this earlier when we began the process of self-examination as a means of better understanding who we are inside. We set our goals so that they are in line with our vision of success. "If I reach my goals, then I will be successful and therefore I will be happy ..." is often how the thinking goes.

The same can be applied to teams. Teams start with goals and a mission. Those goals are connected to a vision of success. For the child-centered team, the thinking might go like this: "We will help the child achieve x, y, z social skills and a, b, c pragmatic speech abilities, and then the team will be successful." There is nothing wrong with these goals and ideas of success. If every team could say that the child met the educational plan, wouldn't the team have been successful? Of course. But often personal perspectives and egos get in the way, and when that happens, the notion of personal success overrides everything else.

It's not our fault that we are so gung-ho on personal success. After all, America was founded through the tenacity and free spirit of young men and women who had a vision of what they wanted their lives to be like and stopped at nothing to go after that. That's how we have been raised and what we have been taught to value. But then we get in a team situation and are told to put these things aside and start using our group skills – all those skills that we have spent little, if any, time thinking about.

How do you think about success? If you are a teacher, you may struggle between running the classroom in the manner that would make *you* look the best versus running it in a way that works for every child in the classroom, including those who require extra care and attention. If you are a parent, you may want to chase professional or personal ideals that would bring you recognition in the eyes of your friends and the outside world but would take you away from investing the one-on-one time that could make the difference between a small gain and a great one for your child.

We have looked at how a team is structured, how it operates, and the key characteristics of effective teams from a technical perspective. But do we know what sort of a person makes a "successful" team member?

What Is Success Anyhow?

What makes a team member "successful" depends on how you define success. Reaching the goals stated on the IEP is one measure of success. Another measure of success is how well the team is functioning. If your team is not working together well, pieces of the plan might be achieved but the overall plan will likely be compromised. You cannot have an effective team with ineffective team members, and you won't have effective team members if they aren't effective as individuals. Assuming they are technically competent, team members' effectiveness starts with who they are on the inside. Who they are as a person will determine what they bring as a team member. There are three essential ingredients to this:

1. Having high integrity

2. Following a process that works

3. Having the right heart-set and mind-set

We have talked about integrity when we discussed core values. Before we see how these work together, let's take a minute to look at the heart-set and mind-set, which is really all about process.

PROCESS

For the team, process is how the IEP gets carried out on a daily basis – how the team members interact, how their skills interlace and build upon each other, and how they work with the child. *What* the team tries to do is to accomplish the goals of the IEP. *How* the goals get accomplished is all about process.

There are two parts to team process. One part you see and the other you don't. The part that you see is how team members communicate and interact with each other. The part that you don't see is the team's mind-set and heart-set. Of course, the team doesn't really have one mind and one heart. But a team culture emerges over time, which can end up influencing individual team members and create a general mood and personality of the team. Ultimately, how you feel and think about other team members is directly related to how you end up treating them.

In the section on understanding yourself, we looked at heart-set and mind-set from a personal level. Now let's look at them as a member of the team and as the whole team.

HEART-SET

Your heart-set is the feelings that you have toward someone or something. If you begin the year with an approach to the teacher that smacks of distrust and neg-ativity, how do you think she will feel? It is true that respect is something that is typically earned. That is, you see a person act respectfully and do respectful things, and she consequently earns your respect. But if you take this wait-and-see approach with the school-based team, it might take three to four months to get to this point. If in the meantime you are questioning, double-guessing, and sending verbal and nonverbal messages that you do not trust or respect the other team members, you could sabotage the team.

This is one of those situations where you may need to take a leap of faith and start off the relationship giving respect freely. This does not mean that you should turn off your antennae and follow blindly. Be alert, be aware, but start off the year giving the team members the benefit of the doubt.

When Harry was entering first grade, his parents were concerned about what kind of teacher he would have. He had just completed a horrific kindergarten year with an experimental combining of two classes of children with special needs. The school team knew that Harry's parents expected the most stellar of teachers given what he had just been through. What they got was Mrs. Powers, new graduate. The first week of school Mrs. Powers sent home Harry's communication journal filled with complaints. Harry's mother immediately went into worry mode and soon began to think Mrs. Powers was not going to be the right "fit." She called the coordinator of special education at the school and explained her concern. The coordinator suggested that Harry's mom sit back and give the teacher a chance. In the meantime, the coordinator also gave a little guidance to Mrs. Powers.

Mrs. Powers ended up being one of the most remarkable teachers Harry ever had. If Harry's mother had gone down that initial negative route towards the teacher rather than put a little trust in her before she truly felt it, she could have ruined the whole year for Harry.

MIND-SET

Your mind-set is the compilation of perceptions and attitudes that you have toward something. For example, when Taku walks into the fourth grade on the first day of school, his teacher groans. She has heard about Taku from his previous teachers, and the news has not been good. Before Taku has done a single thing – good or bad – his new teacher has already formed an impression, which has become an attitude, and a negative one at that.

Like heart-set, it is important that your mind-set be in the right place from the first day of school. You come to school each year with the baggage of the previous year's experiences. You can't help it. But what you can help is what you do with it. Being led by attitudes that were created in a different time and a different place is not fair to this year's team. Most likely you are used to being in a "fighting" mode – fighting for solutions and perhaps services with the school, fighting for cooperation and self-responsibility with your child, and maybe even fighting over it all with your spouse. Lots of negative attitudes can develop, sometimes without you knowing it – self-righteous, self-centered, angry, martyr-like attitudes. Heart-set and mind-set are closely connected. How you feel about someone affects your attitude towards them, and your attitude affects your feeling about them. It doesn't much matter which comes first, heart-set or mind-set, but it is important to realize that each influences the other.

The beginning of the school year is a good time to do a little introspection. Take a look at how you think and feel about the school, the teachers, and the team supporting your child and clean up any bad attitudes and feelings. Maybe you feel you have good reasons supporting the way that you think about the team. It doesn't matter. A good relationship is the backbone of a good team. If you start off with negative attitudes and feelings, the team will never function well together, and thus will not be as effective as it can be.

Let's look at the importance of having a team that works together by examining three camp experiences from one summer.

The summer of Jack's sixth grade, his camp experience was a twenty-five-day program at Kanakuk Kamp, a Christian sports camp. The counselors are of the highest caliber and integrity and are very principled; they want every child to succeed. While they do not have specific training in special needs, they have a desire to understand how they can help each child. In terms of process, the camp is a well-oiled machine, from its mission to the activities that fill each day.

Jack's first camp days were a bit rocky, but I had had several long conversations with the camp director in advance about Jack and had sent a letter with tips for how to best work with him. We had also established an e-mail communication process, and when camp started I provided the counselors with some ideas that helped them settle him in. The twenty-five days were a complete success. Jack came back loving the camp and fundamentally changed.

The second "camp" was an outdoor experience in Utah, run by a science teacher from one of our local schools. There were ten children, most from the school where he taught, and five teachers/counselors. No one knew Jack except for one child. This was only the second year that the program had been in operation, the teacher who was my contact had no background in special needs, and my conversations in advance of the experience (in retrospect) were far too brief. The letter that I had sent with Jack to the airport outlining strategies for working with him never made it into the hands of the counselors until the last day. There were changes to the schedule, a fair amount of free time (meaning unstructured activity – never a good thing for Jack), and an overall loose structure. This was probably a great format for typical children in an outdoor camp experience, but the loose process and questionable competency in terms of working with a child with special needs equaled disaster.

Emerging from the plane after the camp, Jack looked diminished. At first, all I could get out of him were mumbles, which is what happens when things don't go well. Jack had another camp coming up, a basketball camp at a college. I had to determine if he could handle that after the camp. "Let's get cleaned up, dressed up, and go have a great dinner!" I said, and started running the shower water – the likes of which Jack hadn't seen in eight days. At first he refused. Then slowly he got himself ready. Over dinner I heard how children from the school that knew each other started throwing sticks at him. How he joined in and threw some back. How they "interrogated" him until he cracked and finally swore at them. He couldn't take it.

"Doesn't it seem to be a bit of a contradiction to be wearing a cross from Kanakuk and telling someone to go to H-E-double toothpick?" I asked. Jack laughed, knowing how right I was.

"Yes, but I just couldn't take it after a while," came the reply.

Much of the disaster had been my fault. I had not given the teacher enough background information, he had never met Jack in advance of 5:30 a.m. at the airport, and the program did not have the level of structure, supervision, and organization that someone like Jack required. Structure and organization make process. And feeling like the process was out of control, Jack couldn't keep his own process on track.

The last camp for the summer was Michael Jordan's basketball camp. It was a five-day camp held at a nearby college campus. At the camp lots of kids were split into teams and led by high school, college, and NBA players for play/practice all day each day. But the highlight was that you got to see Jordan play for half an hour at the end of each day. When we finally made it to the check-in table, the checker asked Jack, "Any medications?" He knew what she was asking. He was a day camper so, feeling confident that he looked like any other camper, he answered "no."

With that, I slipped the woman an envelope. I wouldn't blow it twice this year – the letter with the tips. I whispered that Jack had some special needs. He saw me and pulled me back from the table.

"You can go now, Mom. There's the door," he said, urging me toward the exit sign. I persisted and made my way to the trainer's table where I had been told to drop off the letter.

At the end of day one – 9:30 p.m. – I went to the door where the kids were to get picked up. No Jack. I looked across the large court and thought I saw Jack heading out the back door.

"Excuse me, sir, where are those kids going?" I asked the security guard who was preventing us from getting on the court (no one gets near Michael Jordan).

Simultaneously pushing the crowd back and waving his hands at me, he said, "Those are the overnighters. They're going back to the dorm."

Oh, great, I thought. The kid can't even figure out what he's supposed to do at the end of the day. There must be five hundred kids in the program. How am I supposed to track him down now? To the dorms I went and searched. No Jack. I returned to the Events Center and found Jack, almost the last one there.

"Where have you been, Mom? I've been waiting here for over thirty minutes." I could nearly see the fumes spilling from his ears.

"I've been here, Jack. Where have you been?" He explained it had taken him a while waiting for a stall in the bathroom. A minor problem of an otherwise good day.

The five-day camp went fine. More than fine. Jack made friends. He loved the basketball camp. He got his picture taken with Jordan. And most important, no behavioral problems. The program was structured, scheduled, and well run. Jack knew what he had to do and where he had to be. No issues.

Why do I take you through all of these stories? To show you the importance that process and people (with the heart-set and mind-set that they bring) play in the experiences of your child's life. Every experience is made up of process and people. For typical children, an incompetent or difficult coach or teacher can be a headache but most can figure out a way to work around it. For the one-of-a-kind child, the coach or teacher is providing a mirror for the child to model himself after. If the mirror isn't clear or doesn't provide the right picture, the child has nothing to follow. How you go through an experience, a day, or a conversation with your child is the journey. The better the preparation, the smoother the journey through life.

IT ALL STARTS WITH REFLECTION

To be the best that you can be – as a person, a parent, a teacher, a mentor, a spouse, a friend, and a team member – begins with knowing who you are and what you want to be. Often, we think in terms of success when we start thinking about what we want to be. That's because we begin to think about goals that we would like to reach.

However, success is a moving target. In fact, the definition of success has changed through the years. Not only does the definition of success change with the times, it changes as we age. In our twenties, we may consider ourselves successful if we get a job and buy a car. By our forties we are beginning to ask ourselves who we are and what we want out of life. If we have reached our level of success, we may say, "Hey, I am successful but am I satisfied?" If we are not successful, we have to face ourselves and wonder why it is that we couldn't reach our goals.

What does a conversation about how we view success have to do with raising a child with special needs? Part of our idea of success has to do with our image of our family. If you have a child who is not what you expected, does that mean that your family is not successful? That you are not successful as a parent? And if so, what does that do to your mind-set, your heart-set, and your core values when you interact with your child and those who are supporting your child on the team?

Understanding and being comfortable with a notion of personal success that is based on core principles, the right heart-set, and the right mind-set will lead to *real* success for you as a person, your family, your child, and the team supporting your child. Remember that old saying, "Where your heart is so are your treasures?" It's not that far from the idea of where you point your sights on success, you will pin your hopes, dreams, energies, heart, mind, and actions.

Getting your idea of personal success in line with your core values, heart-set, and mind-set helps you to become a more effective team member and, in turn, helps to create a more effective team. An effective team member is someone who has high character and standards as well as technical competence, so you need to begin by reflecting on who you are. Without reflection, there is little chance that you will be able to move your inner life along at more than a snail's pace. As you begin to self-examine, think about the process as looking like this:

REFLECTION WHEEL

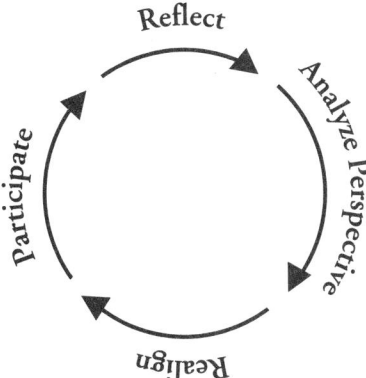

- Reflection – Take stock of your actions, thoughts, and feelings as objectively as you can.

- Perspective – Take a look at what you have discovered in the reflection step more objectively and from a different vantage point than you regularly do.

- Realign – Make some shifts and adjustments in how you think, how you feel, your core values, etc.

- Participation – Get back in and play the game of life with a different heart-set.

MOTHER ALWAYS SAID TO SAY "PLEASE" AND "THANK YOU"

Being part of a smoothly functioning team for your child is like having a healthy body. When we are healthy, we don't think too much about it. But when we are sick, suddenly that is the most important thing in our life. We feel it in every inch of our being, and it takes up much of our thoughts.

Similarly, when the team for your child is working well, it is easy to take it for granted. If your child is in a good phase, you may not think about the team from one IEP meeting to the next. Maybe everything is moving along so smoothly that the team isn't all that necessary.

But if the child runs into issues, or if problems percolate on the team, everything suddenly changes. You will be thinking a whole lot about team and teamwork, desperate to figure out how to get things going in a different direction.

The time and energy that you invest in developing a strong working partnership with the teachers, professionals, staff, and other people who are part of the regular rhythm of your child's daily life is of utmost importance. Although some members of your team may be receiving pay (private doctors, babysitters, etc.), the school-based people get nothing extra for the additional work – and yes, it is additional work – that comes along with serving a child with special needs. What will motivate them? Ideally, your child. That would be good, since he is the key person whom they are serving and the reason that they are coming together. But beyond your child, it is you. You need to be a motivator. Praise them. Thank them. Let them know what a difference they are making in your child's life.

Letting the school team know that you appreciate their efforts can be easy and have huge benefits. It can be as simple as bringing muffins to a meeting, writing a little note of thanks at unexpected times, or just telling the teacher when you notice a gain.

There are other times when you may want to recognize that they have done something extraordinary. For example, the time that Jack lost his retainer. Jack had only had his retainer for two weeks when it got thrown out in the school cafeteria along with his lunch. It was spaghetti and meatballs day. Not a good day for a clear, red, four-inch appliance to get tossed. The lunch room monitor and one of Jack's teachers offered to join my son in the hunt for the hapless retainer. Donning plastic gloves, the three of them turned over the large bin and began searching. Despite their heroic efforts, the retainer was not found.

The next day, I delivered gifts of bath salts to the two teachers with a note that said, "Thank you for going way above and beyond the call of duty."

Teachers go above and beyond the call many times that you see, and many times that you do not see. Be free with your praise, letting them know that you appreciate all they are doing on your child's behalf.

- Four basic ingredients are necessary for a team to be successful:

    1. People of high integrity, having the right heart-set and mind-set

    2. Competent people

    3. A focus or mission

    4. Using a process that works

- People and process are important – they are what make a difference in a child's life.

- By going through the exercise of self-reflecting, you can open up your heart and mind, which will help you to become a more effective team member and, in turn, help to create a more effective team.

SECTION 2

THE FINER POINTS OF PROCESS

An Introduction to Process

An Introduction to Process

Process is about the way that things get done. It is the day-in and day-out preparation, anticipation, interaction, and reaction that is part of everything that we do. When it comes to our children, process is all over the place – from the first breath they take on their life journey to the relationship that we build with them.

Every relationship is a process. The more people who are involved, the more complex the process because of the sheer number of interactions. We have discussed some of the aspects of the process involved in teams, and particularly the key team – the school team. The "how to" is a component of process. In this section we are going to focus on another aspect of process, namely, interaction with the folks supporting your child.

Regardless of what process you are engaged in, interaction is usually a critical component. Where there is interaction, there is communication. Let's begin with communication and examine how powerful it can be in team work.

CHAPTER 1

LET'S TALK ABOUT THAT

The Importance of Good Communication

If someone were to describe you in terms of your communication style, what would they say? Circle a few words or phrases from the list on the following page or add your own. Then write a sentence or two as if someone were describing you.

Communication is the exchange of thoughts, information, and ideas. It is understanding another person's viewpoint and making sure your own viewpoint is understood. Talking without understanding is not communication; it is mere speech. Being an effective communicator is the heart and soul of a good relationship.

A PERSONALITY PERSPECTIVE OF THE TEAM

One way to identify how a team interacts and communicates and how each team member impacts the group is by looking at each team member's personality and style. Of course, what you see on the surface is driven by the heart-set and the mind-set of each person.

From the child's perspective:
- Nagging
- Full of good advice
- Chatty
- Talks to much
- Slow and thoughtful
- "Shotgun Sally"
- Encouraging
- Pushy

If you asked my child to describe my communication style, he would say:

_____

_____

From a fellow team member's perspective:
- She says/does not say what she thinks.
- She begins most of her statements with a negative/She begins most of her statements with a positive.
- She only communicates with the team when there is a problem/She regularly communicates with the team even if there is nothing pressing.

If you asked a fellow team member to describe my communication style, he would say:

_____

_____

Be aware of the impact of personalities. Team morale is a funny thing. It is like quicksand. One wrong move, and everything can change in a heartbeat. Each team member should take a look at the impact that his energy and style has on the team. Manipulators can run away with the meeting and clam others up, quiet ones may not be invested at all, and a gregarious team player may be more interested in getting the other members to like him than accomplishing anything related to the team's goals. If each team member takes responsibility for examining how her personal style impacts the group dynamic and is open to making adjustments if needed, the quality of the team's interactions and work together will rise.

Look at some of the personality types below and see if you recognize any of them on your team. Then see which type you think you belong to and which one you would like to be.

Mr. Negativity – The person who sees the glass as almost drained. He not only finds the flaw but makes the hole bigger in any new idea or brewing issue. He seems to enjoy pointing out the problems rather than looking for solutions. He casts a negative energy over the entire group.

Mr. Optimistic – This is the person who brings a positive spirit and energy the minute he walks into the room. He takes the time and looks for something to rejoice in; not in a fake, Polly Anna sort of way, but in a genuine, caring way. He is the person who takes time to tell a teacher about a story his child told at home that in some way affirms the teacher and her impact on his child.

Mrs. I Know Best – Her superior position can come out as self-righteous, all-knowing, or self-impressed, but no matter how it comes out, it is all about her. A poor listener, Mrs. "I Know Best" talks only to be heard and sees no value in others' ideas or contributions.

Mrs. Open to Suggestions – She never starts out with "We've tried that before" even if the idea has indeed been tried. She might get to that point but not before she has listened without reservation to the thoughts of others. She encourages others to speak their mind and never makes another team member feel belittled or unimportant.

Mr. Secret Agenda – He says one thing but has a different plan in mind.

Mr. Gotta Leave Early – This team member never seems to be fully present. He may be checking his watch or watching the door. You know he isn't really there by the blank stare on his face. He feels that getting to the meeting is more than enough of a contribution and doesn't work much past keeping the seat warm in terms of team interaction and support.

Ms. Talks a Good Game – This is the team member who says all the right things in the meeting. She is supportive of ideas, agrees to take on responsibility, and looks as if she'll be a dependable, contributing member, but once out of the meeting, she does nothing. She talks a good game, but that's the extent of it.

Ms. Chit and Ms. Chat – These two have a running sidebar conversation during the meeting. They make sure that they sit next to each other at all meetings because they need to scribble notes and make comments to each other, and otherwise detract from the meeting.

Mrs. Manipulator – From turning on the charm to weaving the rationale as to why something should be done her way, this team member will do whatever it takes to get things done the way that she wants them done.

Mrs. I've Got Too Much to Do – This is the person who sees special education as one more thing on an already full plate. She may want to do a good job and even be a little interested, but she acts as if the meeting is a waste of her precious time.

How you respond to others is just as important as what you respond with. Your attitude and demeanor, as well as your words, contribute to what kind of team member you are.

COMMUNICATION BASICS

Whether you are with the child or with one of the team members, the same basic rules of being a good communicator hold true. They are as follows:

1. *Be a good listener.* Listen to what the other person is saying. Often we are already interpreting what someone is saying instead of listening to what the person is really saying. Do not try to be a mind reader. Sit back and listen to what the other person feels and what his opinion is.

2. *Try and hear what is behind the words.* Remember that what is being said is only part of the message. Sometimes there is a whole other message behind the words. Listen for it. Look at the person's body language. Ask open-ended questions. Ask feeling questions. Don't assume anything.

3. *Stay open and honest.* It is perfectly fine to have a different point of view or to come from a different perspective. But when that is the case, say so in a non-confrontational way. Conversations can suddenly take U-turns if you begin to play games of manipulation or control. The more you stay in a good heart-set place (see the section on understanding yourself if you need a refresher on how to do this) and communicate from that place, the better the conversation will go and the better the relationship will be.

4. *Be a summarizer.* Have you ever left a conversation and said to yourself, "Now what is it that we just agreed to?" You have no clue what was finally said. Strive for conciseness and closure. Keep in mind what you want to accomplish in your conversation (sometimes you may want nothing more than to try to establish better rapport, and that's fine too!). You may want to say something like this at the end of your conversation so it is clear in the other person's mind as well: "So, just to summarize what we have said here …"

5. *Remember that* how *you say something is as important as* what *you say.* The tone and manner in which you speak (or write) is as important as the content. "I *will* do it right away" has a completely different intonation than if you say, "I will do it right away." The first way of speaking, with an emphasis on *will,* implies that you are agitated or annoyed. The second seems to be a straightforward statement.

FORMS OF COMMUNICATION

There are two kinds of communication, written and spoken. Each represents powerful tools for you, if you use them effectively.

WRITTEN COMMUNICATION

The following is an overview of the most common written forms of communication you should consider using with the school and outside professionals supporting your child.

- *Quarterly (or regularly timed) memos.* These are summary memos written by you or someone that you authorize to do so that provide a snapshot of what is going on with your child from the perspective of the various providers (school, outside therapists, as well as you, the parents) during a specific time period (usually the preceding one to three months). This is an excellent way to bring providers who otherwise often do not see or speak to each other up-to-date on what successes and concerns each has observed as well to give them an idea of how they might build on each other's program. It can also prompt them to contact each other to address specific concerns or opportunities raised in the memo.

Quarterly memos review key issues, outline concerns, highlight strengths and progress, and raise needs that team members would like addressed. Contact information for each team member should be included (with their permission), making it easy for members to get in touch with each other. (A sample memo is provided in Appendix A.)

As mentioned, from my perspective, the parent is the best person to take on the responsibility of writing the quarterly memo. First of all, you are the only person who is in ongoing and direct contact with everyone who is regularly serving your child, both inside and outside of the school, so you are in the best position to ask these people to give you a quick picture of what is going on with your child. You can then coordinate all the information and put it in memo form. If you are not comfortable coordinating information and communicating in writing, find someone who can help you put such a memo together – at least for the first few times until you get the hang of it. Ask the special education coordinator at your child's school, the special education PTA (if your district has one), or a support group if they know anyone who might be available to assist you.

The second reason why it makes sense for you to take on the role of putting out the quarterly memo is that you are ultimately the unofficial team leader for your child. Not the school team leader but your child's Life Team Leader – and these quarterly memos should cover all bases of your child's life, not just his academic progress. While you will be focusing on the IEP goals, be sure to outline issues and progress in other areas that you have been working on, such as general manners, extracurricular activities, and community activities (e.g., learning how to handle a bank account). The more you keep the school advised of what you are working on, the more teachers and other school staff can be partners with you in your efforts.

- *E-mail.* Teachers and school staff are using this form of communication more and more with parents. During the day it is easier for school staff to access e-mail than use the telephone. And it helps parents avoid getting frustrating voice mail messages letting them know that they missed the teacher's call by just five minutes. E-mail is a more convenient method of communication all the way around.

A word of caution, however. The written word is a permanent transcript, so be careful about what you write. Before you push the "send" button, read over what you have written and always ask yourself, "Am I comfortable that anyone could get access to this and know that I wrote it?" If you are frustrated, angry, or upset about something, you may want to set up an appointment and discuss it in person rather than fire off an emotional note that will be committed in writing forever.

- *The daily journal.* A daily journal sent back and forth between the teacher and parents is an excellent communication vehicle that is most often used with younger children. In fact, it is the best way for the parents and the school to stay closely aligned. The daily journal is not the place for you to write your great American novel. It is the place to highlight any outstanding incidents (good or bad), themes that are emerging, concerns, or issues. As your child enters middle school, he will not want to be part of this daily journal concept (it's too embarrassing); e-mail is terrific for children of this age group.

- *The crisis memo.* This memo is written after you have addressed a specific issue in person but want a written record of it. Keep the memo short, concise, and to the facts. In other words, this is not about emotion and your feelings. The memo should outline what the issue is, the discussion surrounding the issue, and what has been agreed to regarding next steps, including actions and deadlines. If unresolved issues remain or if you have concerns that have not been satisfactorily addressed, these should be clearly stated in the memo, but they should not be stated in an aggressive way.

- *The "pat on the back" note.* Not to be undervalued, this is the note that lets someone know that you have noticed her making a difference in your child. It says, "Thank you for caring." It can be accompanied by a small token of appreciation; most often, the note is enough.

When you consider which of these tools is most appropriate for a given situation, you might consider putting into practice what one administrator calls the "twenty-four-hour rule." If you feel the need to write something angry or negative, go ahead and write it out, but then put it away for twenty-four hours. When the time is up, review it and decide if it is appropriate to send. You will often find that you communicated your anger but did not address the problem and potential solutions. You are usually in a better place to do this after your emotions have calmed down and you can look at the matter in a more rational manner.

- *Notes to your child.* Written communication can also be an effective tool to use with your child as he gets older. If you have trouble getting his attention or if you really want to make a point, consider a short note as a way of reaching him. I left the following note one evening after several nights when Jack was "not hungry" at the time I was serving dinner. I thought it might help if he read the words – since he wasn't hearing my words – that I was only serving dinner once and that I did not appreciate eating dinner by myself (Sarah was away at camp and my husband was out of town).

> Dear Jack,
>
> As a matter of fact, no, I do not like eating alone.
> I know it does not bother you. It does me. Try and join me some time.
>
> Love, Mom

This little note got Jack's attention. It even got him to the dinner table a few nights. One little note is not going to turn a kid who has no appetite and therefore no interest in eating dinner at 6 p.m. into a regular dinner partner, but it may make him think. It plants a seed that you can nurture.

SPOKEN COMMUNICATION

Whether we are speaking to children, to colleagues, or to a spouse, there are a few golden rules that we should abide by. Considering that you are setting a tone, and in the case of children, modeling a behavior, how you speak in front of them and to them is how you want them to learn to speak to others. The golden rules are as follows:

1. *Speak with respect.* Notice that I do not say, "Speak as you would like to be spoken to." For one thing, this would not be a meaningful lesson for some children, since the way they might like to be spoken to may not be a way that most people would consider acceptable. Beyond this, since most people understand that respect implies treating others fairly and with decency, it ensures that they will be spoken to in the same manner.

2. *Let it be a conversation, not a lecture.* A conversation implies listening, under-standing, and responding – not just one-sided talking. Be sure that you are practicing all three components of the conversation.

3. *Keep the length of your conversation reasonable.* Parents can get carried away with the details and sagas of their child's issues. Be mindful of what you want to accomplish and what it is that is important for the school or other party to know, and try and stick to that.

4. *Keep your eyes wide open.* Try to understand the world from the unique per-spective of your child. Add to this removing the subjective lens that you automatically view everything from, and you will be much better positioned to understand your child's and others' perspectives.

NEGATIVE SCRIPTS ARE NEVER A GOOD THING

"You shouldn't …," "Why are you … ?," and "If you don't," are examples of an endless array of negative comments. It is easy to get into a habit of using nega-tive dialogue with your child, focusing on all of the things that he is doing wrong. Children with special needs receive many more negative comments than positive comments compared to typical children. Just think about that. For every "Pick up your clothes!" "I told you a thousand times not to pick on your sister!" "If you don't come this minute you will not be allowed to go out later on!" and "Stop tapping that pencil!," there is only a single encouraging "Good job putting away your coat, Jack."

All that negative scripting chips away at the child's self-esteem. Try to implement the 80/20 rule. The 80/20 rule requires that 80 percent of what you say be posi-tive. This can help you go a step further and rethink the way you view mistakes, which will affect the way you think about them and subsequently talk to your child. View mistakes as learning opportunities and worry more about making the child feel worthy and special. By focusing on building self-esteem you will become more empathetic, and your negative scripts will be replaced by more positive ones.

A Little Self-Awareness Goes a Long Way

When you talk, do you listen to how you sound? I'm not talking about whether you are a melodic speaker or a drone (though it is more pleasant to listen to someone who has a varied quality and some modulation to her speech than a flat, monotone speaker). I am talking about *what* you say and the *manner* in which you say it. The next time you have a conversation or you are in a meeting with someone, try to listen to yourself. Afterward, ask yourself these four questions:

1. Was I upbeat and positive in my general tone and manner?

2. Did I wait for the other person to finish speaking before I began or did I interrupt?

3. Did I dominate the conversation or did I speak for a reasonable length of time, giving the other person time to join in with a response?

4. Was I a good listener?

Being a good communicator is a gift. Some folks are born with it. But everyone who wants to can develop it. Communicating when you are seeing eye-to-eye with someone is typically not hard. But what happens when a difference of opinions arises and communication breaks down? How can you and others get through times of difference so that the team doesn't break down in the process? We will address these questions in the next chapter.

- Strive to be an effective communicator. It is the heart and soul of any good relationship.

- Be aware of the impact of personalities on the team. Each team member should take responsibility for looking at how his personal style impacts the group dynamic and be open to making adjustments if needed.

- Find out what form of communication your child's teachers and others working with your child prefer and set up a system to make effective use of it.

- Be conscious of how you come across, not just in your words but in your tone and manner – it is all part of communicating.

CHAPTER 2

WHEN DISHARMONY REIGNS
What to Do When You've Got Conflict

How well would teams function if there were never any disagreements or differences of opinions? If a child met the benchmarks and achieved the goals set in the IEP, his parents would be satisfied, and the teachers, therapists, and school staff would feel good about the work that they were doing with the child. But since we can say with a high degree of certainty (since nothing that our children do is ever predictable, steady, or expected) that everything will not go according to plan, there will be some sticky moments. And that will probably put some pressure on the team.

How the team handles conflict is important to the health of the team. Ideally, the team discussed how conflict will be dealt with way back in the beginning of the life of the team. In fact, how to resolve conflict should be written down as one of the team norms. That way, when conflict does arise, "fighting rules" aren't being made up on the spot, where they may be perceived as being unfair.

Most school administrators and team leaders have participated in some kind of conflict resolution training. Such training usually involves the following four basics steps:

1. Understand and agree on the goal.

2. Share data and information.

3. Ask questions to broaden perspectives to get new ideas and find points of similarity.

4. Find at least three solutions.

The main purpose of any conflict mediation is to get people to move off their specific positions and open up to new ideas and compromises. Often folks get mired in their position and forget the goal. Take the case of Miguel and speech therapy – a real classic.

Miguel is a nine-year-old with Asperger Syndrome who is having difficulty using pragmatic language in social contexts. He has few friends, largely because the only way he knows to communicate with them is to lecture them. Miguel's parents feel that he needs speech therapy four times a week. The school team is recommending that Miguel participate in a speech therapy group once a week with individual therapy once a week. No one is moving off their position.

In this situation, it is easy for everyone involved to forget what is really at stake – helping the child use the language he has to connect appropriately to other children. The amount of therapy is only one component of what must be considered. Issues such as group versus individual therapy, who is in the group, and what kind of group therapy are equally important for Miguel. None of these elements has obvious answers. Only by coming up with a plan, setting benchmarks, and taking data will the team be able to see if two times or four times a week is more effective and what is the best configuration of therapy. In essence, the conflict over the number of times a week for therapy is an argument that doesn't have a known correct answer.

Underlying many conflicts, and probably the one in this example, is emotion. The parents most likely feel that the school team is withholding resources that are rightly theirs, whereas the school may feel that the parents are being unreasonable, only looking for whatever they can get versus what makes the best sense or is reasonable. When perceptions and attitudes like these begin developing, emotions start creeping in, and before you know it, anger and mistrust become part of the conflict equation.

RECOGNIZE YOUR EMOTIONS

One of the most common mistakes people make in trying to resolve conflict is that they approach the issue when they are in a highly charged emotional state. *Nothing* will get resolved if anyone involved in the disagreement is not calm and collected enough to look at the issue objectively.

Emotions are powerful. And anger is one of the most powerful emotions that there is, getting in the way of objectivity and clouding the ability to think clearly, often escalating the very thing that you are trying to get some control over. In order to resolve conflict, it is necessary to do emotional check-ins at every point of the process, as outlined in the following.

RAISE YOUR AWARENESS

Most people don't like conflict, but sometimes it is unavoidable. Rather than look for the common ground or find a way to resolve two viewpoints, we let our emotions take over. You can avoid a lot of conflict by getting better control of your emotions from the start.

Following are some tips to help raise your awareness of how you respond and react in situations that are becoming controversial and to help you control your emotions. Reflecting on these will help you get a better handle on your potentially negative role in conflicts.

- *Know your patterns.* Begin by knowing who you are when you get into controversial territory. When you begin to feel a situation heat up, how do you respond? Can you feel something physical happening to you? Does your pulse quicken, does your stomach turn sour, or do you start sweating? Often physical reactions go along with being upset. If we become attuned to what these are, they alert us to how we are feeling (if our brain has already shut off) and may help us head off at the conflict pass.

You may also have some behavioral reflexes that get in the way of resolving conflict. Are you a runner? Do you leave the scene when things start to heat up so you don't have to deal with the situation? Or do you become defensive, putting the other person off so she is afraid to approach you? Maybe you move right to the blame game, spinning a tale to convince the other person or anyone who will listen why you are not at fault. Or do you just avoid any conflict and vow to get back at the person with some form of retaliation? Knowing what your behavioral reflex is will help you stare it down the next time it steps in the way of conflict resolution.

- *Don't be shy about saying "I'm sorry."* As a kid, I hated saying I was sorry. I would sooner have my mouth washed out with soap than say I was sorry – even if I was in the wrong. It was so hard for me to say those words. But once I got used to saying "I'm sorry," I learned one of the biggest lessons of life: People forgive you and they cut you extra slack. Saying you are sorry is very freeing. It doesn't make you feel smaller; just the opposite, it makes you feel a whole lot bigger: "Hey, I am so secure that I can admit when I am wrong." Saying you are sorry can put the other person in a totally different frame of mind. But don't just take what I say, try it for yourself.

- *Leave the emotion out.* As you begin a disagreement, try to move it to a neutral, non-emotional level. If that's a little unrealistic, how about practicing some good habits like no yelling or raising your voice for starters? If you can train yourself to enter the discussion at a more neutral level, it has a chance of staying focused on problem-solving rather than moving to something emotional that will have little chance of accomplishing anything but only get everyone more upset.

- *Stick to the issue.* You've got plenty to deal with already. There's no need to add fuel to the fire. Stick to the issue before you and try and get it resolved.

- *Learn to monitor yourself.* The next time that you are in a heated discussion with someone, try to stop and look at yourself. Are you keeping your emotions under control? Are you overreacting or under-reacting? Are you getting defensive or closing up? If you catch yourself doing something that could be getting in the way of resolving the issue, STOP. Pay particular attention to your tone of voice. As I told my husband for years, "It isn't what you are saying; it is the tone in which you are saying it."

- *Take a break and rethink it.* When things get too tense, stop, agree to separate, and take a break for however long you need to – ten minutes, an hour, or a day. Once you have cooled off, write down your position and give the supporting information for it. Then do the same for the other person, trying to see things from her position and what she might think supports it. Once you go through this exercise (hopefully the other person has done the same), revisit the issue, sharing what you both wrote. See if you have correctly understood the other person and if she has understood you. In the majority of cases you'll find that you are more open and willing to work towards a solution that suits both of you.

- *Keep listening.* Good listening skills are essential in times of conflict. After the other person has given her opinion, restate what she said to show you were listening and to check if you have it right. (Be sure not to do this in a condescending or belittling fashion.) This ensures that you understand the other person's point of view.

We have spent a lot of time examining how a team might be improved, starting from the heart-set and mind-set of each team member. With all this focus on the self and the team in place, we can now turn to the Life Plan, which is what you hope the team is helping your child work through. This is what Part IV is about.

THE BOTTOM LINE

- Establishing a method for how conflicts will be resolved before they occur saves confusion when a breakdown occurs. This should be done at one of the first team meetings when you are setting team norms.

- Emotions often get in the way of the conflict-resolution process. Until the emotion, often anger, is dealt with, the conflict cannot be resolved.

- You must *want* to resolve the conflict and be willing to see the other person's side before you can seriously discuss the issue at hand. Being open-minded and flexible are prerequisites.

PART IV

THE PLAN

SECTION 1

THE LIFE MAPPING PRIMER

CHAPTER 1

WHEN YOU WORK FROM THE
PHILOSOPHY UP
A Strength-Based Approach

The Life Map is much more than a set of goals and strategies, or the ultimate "to-do list." It is an approach to life that starts with how you view your child. Because the Life Map starts with the child, it was necessary to take a close look at what was going on with him from the inside, as well as with ourselves, which is what we did in the earlier chapters. The more that we see, the more that we understand – and that leads to changing the way that we view the child. Stephen Covey calls this change in our viewpoint a "paradigm shift."[23]

A father is sitting on a train staring out the window, with his four young children circling around him. Literally. They are jumping around on the seats, squealing and hitting each other. The father seems to take no notice. The woman next to him is being jostled and poked until her good humor wears out.

---

[23] Stephen Covey, *Seven Habits of Highly Effective People* (New York: Fireside Books, 1989), p. 29.

"Excuse me, sir, but your children are disturbing me," she leans over to say.

The man pulls himself back from some place very far beyond the windowpane. "Please, I am so sorry. They lost their mother today. We are coming home from the hospital, where they said their good-byes. I am very distracted. I am so sorry," he repeats, and waves the children to come down off the seats.[24]

In an instant, the woman sees the scenario before her in a completely different way. She immediately forgives the children and sees them as lost souls rather than mis-behaved toddlers. The man is a distraught husband and no longer an unaware father. In short, the woman has undergone a paradigm shift. How she viewed the father and children has changed now that she understands the horrific circum-stances they have just come from. All is forgiven. She is tolerant and understanding.

If you want to embrace a true Life Map mentality, you too must be willing to undergo a paradigm shift. The Life Map is not another way to control and con-fine. It begins with understanding the child's diagnosis and problems, and moves quickly on to an understanding of the child's strengths. When you start at a point of asking, "What does this child need to be able to get to his highest potential in life?" you can't possibly look at him from the deficit side. There is no way to look forward if at the same time you are looking back.

To be able to see ahead to as far as you think the child can realistically reach, you must take a growth-oriented approach. According to such an approach, the child and the process are organic, capable of change; in fact, they are in a constant state of change. Adopting this approach involves a paradigm shift of the mind-set and heart-set. Now do you see why we had to do all of that pre-work?

THE STRENGTH-BASED APPROACH OF THE LIFE MAP

The shifts that we explored in the section on understanding yourself and your heart-set, mind-set, and self-set are consistent with the strength-based model underlying the Life Map. They call for you to coach, mentor, and teach using positive reinforcement – building on strengths, drawing out what is already there, and remaining focused on the idea that the child will grow and develop through skill development and learning.

---

[24] This story is taken from Stephen Covey, *Seven Habits of Highly Effective People* (New York: Fireside Books, 1989), pp. 30-31.

The Life Map approach encourages playfulness and joy. When you are looking for ways to raise a child up, there is a sense of possibility and hope. When you are taking an approach of controlling through consequences and punishments, there is friction in the air. Fill out the following to see what approach you may be using.

POSITIVE OR NEGATIVE?

When you come across the child doing something that he is not supposed to be doing, what is your reaction most of the time? (Check all that apply.)

_____ Anger

_____ Frustration

_____ "Where is the reward system plan?"

_____ "I need to control this."

_____ "What consequence makes sense here?"

_____ "Hey, what he's doing is wrong!"

_____ "I need to talk to the team about correcting this behavior."

_____ "He's probably trying to get my attention."

_____ "I think he may be manipulating me."

_____ "If doing the right thing doesn't matter to him, it doesn't matter to me either."

_____ "I can't have any conflict here. What can I do to keep this from happening again?"

If you checked off more than one statement, you should be congratulated for being honest. It is very, very difficult not to have these types of reactions when your child is throwing a tantrum because he can't watch the next television program (he's already watched five shows in a row), he doesn't want to come to dinner, or his brother took the color car he wanted for *Monopoly*. Unfortunately, none of these statements is in line with the Life Map attitude.

Let's try to reframe some statements you might typically use into a Life Map-friendly way of thinking. In fact, let's go one step further and look at them from several viewpoints.[25]

Viewpoint	Deficit-Based, Traditional Approach	Strength-Based Approach of Life Map
Different views of the child	He's doing that on purpose!	He is having trouble with impulsivity.
	He could control himself (he has the skills), but he doesn't want to.	He doesn't have the skills that he needs to control himself.
	He has no motivation. He doesn't care.	We need to encourage him. He's given up.
Different mind-sets you could have	I have to control that bad behavior.	Let me reinforce what he's doing right.
	There! He's made a mistake.	What can I do to help him get going in the right direction?
	What consequence can I give him so he won't do this again?	What can I teach him from this?
	I can't let a meltdown happen again. I have to figure out how to stop them.	Okay, so he had a meltdown. What did we learn so we can give him some tools to try and avoid this in the future?

The deficit-based approach seeks compliance as a means of changing behavior. Certainly, consequences have their place, but if your whole basket of tricks is consequence based, you may not be changing behavior for the long haul. You may be getting only short-term compliance necessary for the child to stay out of perceived trouble.

---

[25] Taken from *A Strength-Based Approach to Treatment*, Andrew L. Reitz, Ph.D., Child Welfare League of America, 2 Adams Place, Suite 305, Quincy, MA 02169, areitz@cwla.org. Reprinted with permission.

The Life Map approach, on the other hand, by focusing on building strengths and skills, acknowledges that there will be more bumps and stumbles along the way because you are deliberately allowing more mistakes to occur. But, in a way, you have to. This is the time to work on developing key competencies, and to do so the child needs practice, practice, practice. If children with social and behavioral challenges are not allowed to fail and to learn that failing is okay, how will they get through the infinite range of new social skills and nuances that are demanded at each developmental level? Helping children to learn how to utilize their strengths and ever-growing basket of skills to face new predicaments and challenges is the process orientation of the Life Map.

The ideal time to work on developing competencies is when the behavior that needs reinforcing occurs. For example, if you are working on sharing, the time and place to focus the child on the concept is right before his play date – don't leave it to the Thursday social skills group and think that you have covered teaching this skill. The skill must be taught at the place and time that it is needed. If little Sean is learning how to share, the playground monitor should remind him to take turns right before he leaves the cafeteria to go to recess. The monitor should then observe his behavior and share her observations with his classroom teacher, who can talk to him right away about any behaviors that weren't consistent with good turn-taking or conversely, praise and reinforce good behavior. Right away, with a real-time example, Sean can see what didn't work and learn accordingly. The more you teach "in the moment," cueing the child before the activity and reviewing and reinforcing his performance after the event, the more he will learn to self-monitor and train himself to utilize the desired skills in each setting.

ARE YOU GETTING IT?

Look at the list of options below and circle the one in each pair that you think is more important.

WHAT IS MORE IMPORTANT?

The cake	Making the cake
Riding the bike	Buying the bike
Your birthday present	Your birthday

If you circled any of the answers on the right-hand side, you are seeing the process. Those on the left are the goals, the endpoints. The cake may taste great, riding the bike is a thrill, and who doesn't love a present? But these are the goals, and if it turned out you didn't like the cake flavor, the bike didn't work, or the present wasn't what you wanted, it would all have been a waste. But if you had focused on the process part of each of these – the experience of the day or the event – you would probably still have found something to sing about even if the payoff wasn't quite what you had imagined. Such is a process orientation.

Now look at the pairs below and circle the one in each pair that appeals to you more.

Which Role Appears To You?

Encourager	Controller
Supporter	Evaluator
Teacher	Disciplinarian

Okay, that was a dead giveaway. You would have had to be sleeping through this section not to realize that the roles on the left are those that any Life Map, strength-based team player would focus on. Those on the right are what we often assume when we feel that the child and life are not going as smoothly as we would like them to.

In the Life Map model, children (as well as parents and teachers) learn to view mess-ups and failures as opportunities to learn. Rather than focusing on extinguishing a given behavior, the Life Map concentrates on teaching children what tools they need to be able to manage themselves so that they have the personal control to prevent such situations in the future. Everything is an opportunity to work on a competency and gain a skill in the Life Map model.

- In order to embrace the Life Map model, you must be willing to undergo a paradigm shift to your heart-set and mind-set.

- The Life Map model uses a strength-based approach, focusing on what skills and competencies the child needs rather than squaring off on his problems.

- The Life Map approach calls for parents and teachers to coach, mentor, and teach using positive reinforcement – building on the strengths, drawing out what is already there, and remaining focused on the idea that the child will grow and develop through skill development and learning.

CHAPTER 2

The Nuts and Bolts of Life Mapping
Getting Started

I f you think that life is one of destiny, you won't buy into the Life Mapping concept because, according to that world view, things just happen and it all works out as "it is supposed to" in the end. But if you believe that you have a lot to do with how life turns out, stick with me. In fact, if you believe that you have a lot to do with who you become and that you have a lot of influence on who your child becomes, Life Mapping is for you.

Why Our Children Need a Life Map
Life Mapping is a process of intentionally and thoughtfully creating a roadmap to become who you want to be. When our children are young, we do this for them rather automatically. But once the teens hit, parents' beliefs, values, and any opinions offered are either flatly rejected or politely ignored.

This is a normal and natural part of growing up, and it is why parents and teenagers often butt heads. Teens try on different personalities, styles, and perhaps even values, in an effort to find out who they are and determine who they want to be. If my thirteen-year-old typical teen daughter ever thought that I had something called a Life Map for her, even one that was only in my head, she would rebel against anything it contained. With typical children it would be a little odd for you to be setting their vision anyway. They usually set their own. You will stand on the sidelines, guiding and probing, seeking to influence it a bit here or there but, by and large, they have the necessary tools to move ahead on their own. It is part of the growing-up process for them to figure out who they are and who they want to be.

But for a child who has neurological and similar compromises, the teen years can be full of pitfalls. Depending on his level of functioning, he may think that he has all the same abilities as his typical peers, although in reality his cognitive or emotional abilities may lag behind his chronological age. Leaving him to his own devices does not help him acquire the skills that he lacks.

As his parent, you cannot simply stand aside and let the developmental stages take their course. Your child may have been able to modulate some behaviors, even extinguishing some, but the engine behind these behaviors is still in motion. Your child may have learned to share, to use "good" language, to not interrupt, and other basics of social interaction, but at each stage, there are new social challenges on the outside and the same old cognitive engine on the inside.

Tom, a twelve-year-old with ADHD and PDD, was excited about starting to play football. He had wanted to play for a long time, but his parents had worried that his impulsivity and self-orientation would reign and that he would be too rough on the field. When he turned twelve, they finally decided that Tom was as ready as he would ever be for the game.

Before the first practice Tom invited two boys from his class over after school. His mother thought this was a good idea, since she didn't know how to help her son put on the equipment. She gave the boys a snack when they arrived home and sent them upstairs to Tom's room to change. A while later, the two boys came down and went outside, leaving Tom to his own devices. Tom's sister, Peggy, ran down the stairs after the boys to find out where they were going.

Soon, she returned to the kitchen. "Mom, you have got to have a talk with Tom!" Peggy said. "He put on one of those cup things and was walking around banging it and saying inappropriate things. Even the boys were grossed out. That's why they went outside."

In this story the outcome was more or less harmless. Tom's mom asked his father to talk to him about the situation, and Tom no longer turned his athletic supporter into a joke. Tom's impulsive comments are more under control than when he was seven, but they have not disappeared just because he is older. He will need guidance and modeling for years to come.

Our children can be trained in appropriate responses for specific situations, be taught systems of thinking that will help them with self-control and social decision-making, and, when appropriate, use medication that can target symptom relief. But their underlying disorder generally will not disappear. Life Mapping creates a more deliberate environment, which reduces the barriers that can trip the child up and creates opportunities for teaching, training, and practicing newly acquired skills.

It is important that your child not feel that his world is being completely manipulated. He must be made a partner in the process and have some control over it, although parameters and a structure should be present to support him and to prevent him from falling back on the natural instincts that may be limiting him. Your child may not have the interest or self-determination to be an avid participant when you think he is ready to be, but in becoming part of the process, he will eventually gain enough skills to realize that ultimately it is up to him to continue on his own journey.

What, Exactly, Is the Life Map?

Your personal Life Map is a roadmap that keeps you oriented on the path that connects where you are at that moment with where you want to be. It is the strategies, guidelines, and activities that you hope will lead you toward the vision you have set for yourself. Until your child is able to be a part of this process for his own life, you and those who you believe understand him and have his best interests at heart will need to develop this for him. Though he may not be a part of the formal planning process in his younger years, understanding your child, his interests, passions, limitations and strengths, will allow him to stay front and center of the Life Map.

Even if it's just one or two people who set the vision, the roadmap developed to support the vision is only as effective as the people who are involved in the trip. In the case of your child, in the years before his cognitive functioning allows him to be part of this process, you and your spouse (or other significant family members or care providers) will be the ones developing the vision (hopefully with input), but it is the people who are working and interacting with your child on a daily basis who will be most effective in carrying out the steps that will help bring about that vision. As your child gains skills, insights, and reasoning ability, it is critical that you make him part of the process. This doesn't need to be any more formal than conversation in a quiet place when you think he is "in the mood" to do some reflecting. The more he is part of developing the vision, the more he will be a willing participant in carrying it out.

There are five levels to developing the Life Map. It starts with the most global view of where you want your child to be and works down to specific actions.

Vision							
Mission				Mission			
Goal #1		Goal #2		Goal #1		Goal #2	
Strategy #1		Strategy #2		Strategy #1		Strategy #2	
Tactic #1	Tactic #2	Tactic #1	Tactic #2	Tactic #1	Tactic #2	Tactic #1	Tactic #2

VISION

A vision is the picture of the future that defines what you seek to become. It is what you hope to be when you have reached your potential. In terms of your child, it is the loftiest ideal you can imagine for him within the bounds of what is reasonable. It's easy to see visions in concrete things such as products:

• McDonald's: To be the most profitable fast-food restaurant in the world.

• The New York Yankees: To be the number one team in major league baseball.

Why is a vision important for the Life Map?

First, having a vision, and not just a dream that you write down and never look at again, ensures that you are working on the right things.

Second, articulating a vision forces you to be intentional; that is, to think reflectively on what should be in your vision for your child. For example, is having your child be a person with a faith base important to you? If "having an active faith" is part of your vision but you haven't built any activities into your family life to promote the child's spiritual base, you will never reach the vision. So which is inconsistent? The faith statement or failing to take the necessary actions to get there? By forcing yourself to think through what is truly the vision for where you want your child to be you illuminate such inconsistencies.

Third, having an articulated vision ensures that everyone who is on the team or closely involved with your child's life is on the same page. Certainly, many parents and teams operate with no more than an IEP and the child makes progress. An IEP has visions, goals, and strategies, which is excellent. But it does not always encompass the whole child. You might think of the Life Map as an IEP on steroids. It is that much bigger and stronger, and that is because it incorporates the whole child and every part of his day.

An example of a vision statement for your child (let's call him Barney) might look something like this:

BARNEY'S VISION STATEMENT

Barney will lead a life of happiness in a way that is satisfying to him and is a positive contribution to those around him

OR

Barney will reach the highest academic, social, and personal levels that he is capable of, in a way that utilizes his talents and minimizes his limitations, so that he will be a responsible, capable, and principled person with a satisfying sense of purpose and joy of life.

This vision statement will look different depending on your child's current level of functioning and an assessment of what he may be able to grow to. There is an aspect of expectation in the vision statement. You expect that your child will be able to attain the vision set forth. It is senseless to put forth some lofty vision statement that you know, deep down, your child will never be able to attain.

What if the vision statement for your child read something like this: "Olivia will be a child protégé in piano, known throughout the United States?" You write this, but the child is already seven years old and has not yet taken a single piano lesson. Not such a realistic vision when you really look at it, is it? The vision statement must have, in the estimation of those who have developed it, a reasonable chance of being attained.

Because some children do not have a steady or consistent rate of development, it is sometimes difficult to imagine what is a reasonable stretch. Don't worry. While the vision statement is not something that should be changed weekly, or even yearly, it is not set in stone either. It should be your best guess for the next long haul. If your child is seven, the vision statement should be geared to young adulthood, but should be assessed and adjusted, if needed, at each developmental stage – pre-adolescence, adolescence, and so on.

While every piece of the Life Map is critical, if this first level, the vision, is off, then everything else that follows will be askew. Take your time in carefully thinking through the vision to be sure you are on the right track.

Ideas for the Vision
To help you get started developing the vision for your child, complete the following exercise.

WHAT'S IN THE VISION?

Circle all the words that reflect what you feel should be in your child's vision statement, and add others that come to mind.

Happiness	Resilience	Community oriented	_____
Self-worth	Sense of purpose	_____	_____
Self-acceptance	Connectedness	_____	_____

Use two or three of the words you circled as the lynch pins of the vision statement. Be wary of picking a few from each column. If you do that, the vision will end up lacking focus and be too global to hold any personal meaning for you and your child.

The Vision Statement in Simple English
In simple terms, the vision for your child might include these sorts of things:

- To be happy – A feeling of well-being, satisfaction with life, comfort, peace, and tranquility.

- To be resilient – Able to effectively deal with whatever comes his way, including disappointments and failures, and still feel good about himself.

- To have a right heart-set – Positioning the heart to be accepting; valuing others and seeing them as worthy. Without the right heart-set, we have no motivation or interest in connecting with anyone else.

- To be principled – To act in accordance with personal principles. I call this your authentic self.

- To have the skills and competencies necessary to lead a responsible life.

MISSION

The mission is the specific accomplishment needed to realize the vision. Some examples of missions include the following:

- McDonald's: To offer a high quality of food and an unsurpassed level of customer service.

- The New York Yankees: To have strong pitchers, players with a combined batting average of .325, and a tough outfield.

The missions for the child in the above vision statement example might look like this:

BARNEY'S VISION STATEMENT
MISSIONS

- Barney will graduate from college or complete enough education to gain and maintain a job that gives him personal satisfaction.
- Barney will develop and maintain healthy relationships.
- Barney will be self-supporting.

Try to look at each aspect of your child – academic, social, emotional, and spiritual – and determine what the mission would be in each area. Think of the Life Map as the mega plan, encompassing all aspects of the child's life. The more specific you can be for each aspect, the easier it will be to establish goals. While goals will be developed as part of the IEP for your child's educational dimension, this is just one part of the larger Life Map. Assuming that the social, emotional, and spiritual aspects of your child are just as important as the academic (and they should be), your missions for your child in these areas should be just as well thought out and pursued as the IEP.

GOALS

Goals are what needs to be achieved in order to reach the missions. Goals reflect the missions and vision for your child. A well-conceived goal includes the following three elements:

1. *Specific* – You should have a clear sense of what needs to be done to accomplish the goal. For Jack, "Being able to have a play date that is safe, interactive and enjoyable for Jack and his friend" is a far better goal than "Jack will have fun with friends." Saying "fun" without defining it is too vague and provides no direction.

2. *Measurable* – You should be able to determine when and how a goal is reached. There are a number of ways to measure a goal, from direct observation to formal evaluation. In the play date example, observing what happened during the children's time together will provide you the data that you need to assess if the play date met its goals.

3. *Time bound* – A goal should have a specific completion date. Making it open-ended to be achieved "whenever" leaves it open to never getting accomplished. Obviously, with the play date there is a specific period of time that you can review.

STRATEGIES

Strategies are ways to accomplish the goals. You have many options to choose from. In selecting a strategy, look at the strengths, interests, and needs of your child, get the team's input and opinions, and select the strategy that best suits your child. In the play date example, one strategy is to set up an activity that interests both boys and involves taking turns.

TACTICS

Tactics are the very specific steps that must be implemented to support the strategies. Usually, there are multiple tactics supporting each strategy. For the play date, you could take the boys bowling or teach them how to play a new board game, for example.

FROM ONE TO MANY

When the Life Map is built, it resembles a pyramid (see page 152), with one single vision at the top supported by one or two missions, several goals, multiple strategies supporting each goal, and whatever number of tactics necessary to accomplish the strategies.

BUILDING BLOCKS OF THE LIFE MAP

Your diagram may look slightly different from this one, depending on the number of goals you set and the number of strategies and tactics you develop to support those goals, but all of these levels must be incorporated into the Life Map for your child, and they should all stem from just one global vision.

THE LIFE MAPPING ATTITUDE

The big day has arrived for the McRae family's annual vacation. This is the most anticipated time of the year. It is the one time when the craziness of running in too many directions is put aside, and the family can enjoy each other's company. This year they have planned a trip to the Grand Canyon. For months, Mom and Dad have been preparing the kids for the trip; they have gone whitewater rafting at a local river so that they will be ready for the bigger whitewaters of the Colorado River. They have read books and seen an IMAX movie about the Grand Canyon. Mom has made all sorts of reservations at the park, from riding down the canyon on donkeys to securing rooms at the only hotel in the park – a feat in and of itself.

In the morning before leaving, Mom makes sandwiches and Dad does a quick run to the gas station to check the oil and tires and to gas up. The kids argue about who is going to sit where, until Mom assigns the seats – and that's that. Everyone is finally in the car, ready to go. Dad turns around with the map in his hand and shows the family where the park is.

"That's where we'll be fifteen hours from now!" Dad says, checking his watch. He turns on the radio and puts on the station of choice for the first hour of the trip. (The

THE NUTS AND BOLTS OF
LIFE MAPPING

kids have decided to take turns choosing which station they will listen to.) Seatbelts are snapped and off they go.

The highway is clear and the family's van is cruising along for the first four hours. Mom suggests that they all play the Alphabet Game and the kids are nicely occupied looking for things outside that start with the letter A.

"I think I'm going to be carsick," five-year-old Ben says suddenly. Mom turns around, and sure enough, Ben is as white as a ghost. Before another word is said, Dad has pulled off the road and Ben is out the door and, good to his word, becomes sick to his stomach. Everyone piles out; Dad keeps the other children occupied while Mom figures out what to do with Ben. She decides his motion sickness was probably caused by Ben's earlier reading (reading always makes him carsick), so the family hustles back in the car and continues on their way – no more reading for Ben.

It's time for Sally's turn to pick the radio station; she picks an Oldies station. Before long, everyone, including Dad, is singing to the Supremes and has forgotten the Ben detour. They are supposed to spend their first night in a small town outside of Fort Collins, but since they made such good time Dad suggests they show the kids the capital of Colorado, so they push on to Denver. Phone calls are made, reservations changed, and soon they arrive in Denver. The family enjoys a wonderful, spontaneous visit to the city's aquarium.

In the morning they wake up to the sound of thunder. Dad looks out the window to see that it is indeed raining – pouring buckets to be exact. It'll be a long day, he knows. Once on the road, the driving is as bad as Dad had feared. Worse, in fact. Although they have only two more hours to go, it takes them seven hours. And the rain gets worse and worse.

Finally, at dusk, they arrive. Dad pulls the van into the turn that indicates the way to the Grand Canyon's entrance. But when he gets to the booth to get their park entrance tickets, they are met with a sign saying "Park closed due to flooding. Stay tuned to AM 1010 for park updates." The kids complain, Mom groans, and Dad gets out of the car into the pouring rain to find a park ranger in the nearby office.

When he returns, the news is not good. "They expect the park to be closed for at least two or three days," he reports in a low voice. That was exactly the length of time they *were planning to stay at the park. No one says anything for a full five minutes. When someone finally breaks the silence, it is Mom.*

"We can sit around and complain or we can do something about this. We want to go to a national park, right? Let's put our heads together and pull out the map and see what else we can come up with. We are all disappointed, but if we let this get to us we'll have a miserable time. Let's pretend we are explorers!" Dad takes his cue from Mom, and before long they have decided to head to Yosemite Park. Dad turns the van around, and Mom starts making phone calls to hotels. The vacation will be a success.

Let's take a look at how the Life Map was operating in the McRae family. The *vision* that Mom and Dad McRae have set for their family is to be a family that enjoys a loving, fun, and healthy relationship. One of the *goals* to achieve that vision is to spend time together as a unit. The *strategy* was to go on one family vacation a year. And the *tactic* was to go to the Grand Canyon.

Lucky for the little McRaes, Mom McRae had internalized the family vision. When disaster struck, she knew that staying calm and positive was important to keep the mood and energy of the family going in the right direction. She knew that they could still have fun and share experiences; they would just be different experiences than what they had planned.

The Life Map keeps you in a proactive rather than a reactive mode. Because life is always changing and because people constantly change, it is impossible not to have unexpected situations arise, even when you have a carefully mapped-out plan. But when the unexpected comes, you will be in much better shape to decide how you want to respond and what action you want to take if you have some endpoint in mind. If the McRaes hadn't been mindful of the fact that the point of the vacation was to be together, they might have turned around and driven home. The specific goal was to get to the Grand Canyon, but that was only one of any number of options available to serve a higher goal or vision – to foster a loving family.

In Real Life, the Life Map Can Be More Informal

The McRaes didn't sit there like the Stepford Family and work their way through some articulated Life Map that was pinned to the refrigerator door. And you shouldn't expect to have to do that either. Like most of us, you probably go through your finances or insurance program once in a while to make sure it is meeting your family's current needs. The Life Map is the same sort of thing. You take a day once in a while, think it all through and come up with the general outline for a plan. Depending upon your personality type, it can be as detailed as you would like. Don't get all strung out on the details. Focus upon the basics and the big ideas. Speaking of big ideas, let's take a closer look at goals.

THE BOTTOM LINE

- Even if your child has overcome or modulated some behaviors, his disorder is still there. At each stage of a child's life, there will be new social challenges. Life Mapping helps create a more deliberate environment to remove barriers and put in more opportunities for training and teaching the needed skills.

- Life Mapping begins with a vision of who and what your child can be from the loftiest view possible, taking his strengths and limitations into account. As he gets older, involve your child in this exercise to the degree that his level of functioning and cognitive abilities will allow.

- Life Mapping includes the missions, goals, strategies, and tactics that you hope will lead your child to the vision that together you and your child create for him.

CHAPTER 3

Unfolding the Tent

Helping a Child Reach His Potential

Developing a long-term vision – that rather lofty, global statement that we looked at earlier – is great, but if that's the only thing you have in front of you, it is too far in the distance and too big a leap from where your child is today. By backing up and thinking about the specific accomplishments that are necessary to reach that vision, you can begin to formulate plans, which we can think of as the missions, that are more realistic for a nearer timeframe. When you develop these missions, think about them in terms of immediate (within one year), medium-term (one to three years), and longer-term (five years) blocks of time.

The immediate missions are those that you think your child has a reasonable chance of reaching within one year. These should all be reflected in goals, strategies, and tactics for the coming year. The medium-term missions are those that you feel fairly comfortable that your child will be able to achieve in one to three years if he continues at his current rate of progress. Include at least one stretch –

something that is a long shot, not impossible but something that will not be easy for the child to reach, given his current functioning level. After all, you never really know how far he can go if you don't raise the bar a little. Finally, the longer-term missions are those that require guesstimating what you think your child can accomplish within five years.

Let's see how this spins out, using an example of one aspect of our family's Life Map.

A LONG-TERM MISSION

One of the elements of our *vision* for both of our children is that they have a strong sense of spirituality. One of the *immediate missions* to reach this vision, since they were toddlers, has been for them to have peer experiences in settings that promote this development. One *goal* we set in this area, even before the children were old enough to attend, was for Jack and Sarah to attend Kanakuk Kamp, the oldest Christian sports camp in the country. You need only spend a few minutes at the camp to understand why it has been the touchstone for thousands of children for over thirty years.

For Sarah, we were able to stay right on track. This summer will be her seventh at the camp. But with Jack, we knew that some things had to change. Not the *vision*; we felt that he needed a spiritual base as much as anybody. And not the *mission* – although it became a five-year mission for Jack instead of a one- to three-year mission. The goal was still to get him to Kanakuk. Our *strategy* was to first get him successfully through other camp programs with the level of support that would prepare him for some day attending Kanakuk. Our *tactic* was to find the best camp for Jack to do this (which took several years and many mistakes) and then work with the camp and Jack to help him gain the organization and transition skills he would need for a typical camp.

To appreciate what happened means you have to know how Sarah began her career at Kanakuk. When Sarah was six years old, she spent her first summer at Kanakuk Kamp.

Sarah didn't know a soul that first year, but she had an adventuresome spirit. When we arrived at the Springfield, Missouri, airport after twelve hours of traveling, Sarah immediately spied the big bus that would take her and the other campers who were arriving at the same time to the camp, ninety miles from the airport. She turned to me as I was coming off the escalator from the arrival flights and said, "There's the bus. I'm all set. You can go home now." I was stunned – and torn between being proud that she felt so confident and hurt that she didn't even seem to mind leaving me. I took her cue and retraced my steps to the gate that would take me on the first leg of my journey home.

If Jack could make it to Kanakuk, it would be exciting for two reasons. It would mean that he was able to manage himself well enough to be there with typical children and that he might have an experience that could significantly impact his life. I tucked these thoughts away and didn't think about them again.

Year after year Sarah went to Kanakuk. Jack went to overnight camp, too. Once we had lived through several camp disasters in our area and had found the right camp for Jack, he finally had a powerful seven-week experience. The camp worked closely with us and with Jack's school, developing behavioral and social goals. Although the camp's days were filled with typical camp activities, from water play to basketball, the counselors were very much on top of the behavioral goals as well.

As mentioned earlier, in the fall of Jack's fifth-grade year, I began to think about his options for middle school. As I thought this through and talked to his teachers, I began to understand that our son had made some significant behavioral gains in the last two years. Out of my brain popped the word *Kanakuk*. Could he do it? Was he ready? We decided to go for it.

On June 26, Jack and I arrived at the Springfield, Missouri, airport, having joined several kids on the connecting flight in Chicago who were also headed for Kanakuk. Jack had noticed that a number of children getting on the flight were traveling alone. As the plane got closer to Springfield, Jack began to ignore me. And by the time the airplane doors opened and we were walking into the terminal, I had all but lost him. I watched as he marched up to a woman wearing a Kanakuk tee shirt and holding a clipboard. She pointed to where the buses were, and he took off.

"Jack!" I yelled, running to catch up to him. I stopped about six feet from him and he turned around. "Aren't you even going to kiss me good-bye?" I asked.

With a twinkle in his eye, he looked at me and said, "No," waved his hand, and turned to join the other kids already lining up for the bus. I was forgotten immediately.

I stayed in close touch with the director of the camp via e-mail and telephone the first few days that Jack was at Kanakuk. They were a bit rocky as Jack adjusted to the requirements and expectations of a "real camp." We brainstormed. The director relayed more information and some suggestions to Jack's counselors. By day five I was breathing easy. Jack had settled into the program.

Jack's first letter to us said it all:

Dear Mom and Dad,

I am loving camp. Please find out if I can go every term next year. I caught a lizard today. I have been down every rope slide except one. Can you send my baseball glove, reptile book, and 300 water balloons?

Love, Jack

A SHORT-TERM MISSION

On a much more everyday level, and extremely fundamental to leading a successful life, was the mission that had been on Jack's list for ages of turn-taking. Jack had very little of this as a young child. One part of our *vision* for him is that he have satisfying relationships. This I was determined that he'd achieve, even at the age of five when he had absolutely no interest in interacting with anyone unless they were slimy green and croaked. The *mission* was to get him interested in interacting with another peer. The *goal* was to work on his ability to demonstrate self-control. Of course, this was decidedly tricky, if not impossible, for a child with ADHD. The *strategy* was to put him in situations where he would be required to wait his turn. I would have to be sure that there was a reasonable amount of time for waiting and not place unrealistic expectations on him. The *tactics* included playing board games with him at home, teaching him and his sister how to play chess, enrolling him in an after-school chess club, and having the speech and occupational language therapists work turn-taking into their therapy.

Taking turns was coming at Jack from all sides. The message was loud and clear. "Hold your horses, it's my turn!" was my frequent response when we started the board-game approach. A few months later I started to see small changes, particularly in chess, where the rules were very precise, down to using a clock we each punched to indicate when our turn was over and it was the other person's turn. Jack was learning the rhythm and rules of sharing. He couldn't avoid it. The message was everywhere.

And that is the strength of the Life Map. It reinforces the goals in all aspects of the child's life.

LIFE SKILLS

As you work your way along the Life Map, you are helping your child build competencies, skills, and strengths in three general areas:

1. *Practical competencies.* These can be anything from getting dressed, brushing teeth, and looking respectable in the morning to learning how to manage time and balance a checkbook. While you might be able to show a typical child these things once and feel confident that she will master or at least know how to go about mastering these simple daily duties, for an exceptional child it can take months of work before the child is convinced that this is something that he should do.

2. *Technical competencies.* Whether your child should or will be able to attend school beyond high school is something that you will figure out with the team and your child.

3. *Relationship competencies.* No matter how complex your child's challenges are, he will be relating to others in his life at some level. The better he can function in the world, the more he is seen as competent and valued for his contributions. This is true on many levels. On a practical level, he needs to be able to make a transaction at the bank, get through the grocery store, and buy a pair of shoes. On a personal level, he has to be able to connect to colleagues, his superiors, and those who work under him. And it would be our dream of dreams for him to have good friends. All of this takes the ability to read cues, share feelings, and be sensitive, dependable, reliable, and trustworthy, for starters. In fact, developing a healthy mind-set, heart-set, and core values will be the foundation for your child to develop relationships.

The extent to which the child is developing all these competencies is, in large part, determined by what is modeled for him and what he is encouraged to practice, in addition to his potential. And this is where the team, in the broadest sense of the word, comes into play. As discussed earlier, anyone who is regularly interacting with your child may be thought of as being part of the team. These are people who have an opportunity to build a relationship with your child and, in so doing, can teach him what he will not be able to pick up on his own. This doesn't happen through osmosis. Instead, the Life Map has a way of teaching that is built into it by its very nature.

STATE EXPECTATIONS

The role model/teacher/coach must be very clear with the child in terms of what is expected of him. The child should be conscious of the immediate goals of the Life Map. These are the only things that are relevant to the child. Not the medium- or longer-term goals, and certainly not the vision. For him, what matters is what affects his life today. Briefly, and specifically, let him know what you are working on.

MODEL BEHAVIOR

I always tell coaches and instructors who have not worked with Jack before that it will be far more useful to get out and show Jack how to do something than to lecture. Jack is a visual processor. Think about how your child takes in information best and encourage those who are working with him to deliver the strategies in a way that suits his learning style (such as auditory or experiential).

Modeled behavior has the potential of sending a strong message. But this only happens if the child respects and admires the person who is doing the modeling. Naturally, you have to earn respect first. The child will probably not make a leap of faith and follow your lead if he does not feel supported, encouraged, cared for, and listened to, and if his own opinion is not respected.

PREPARE FOR PROBLEMS

There will be problems. Stop thinking that life will one day be perfect when you stop the problems from occurring, the tantrums from happening, and the mess-ups from messing up your life. This is one of the paradigm shifts that you have to make.

You can't avoid the problems, but you can do a better job of anticipating them. The more that you can anticipate, the more you can adjust the environment and prepare the child for what lies ahead.

KEEP ACCENTUATING THE POSITIVE, TEACH FROM NEGATIVE EXPERIENCE

The child must feel that it is okay to make a mistake or encounter a problem and that you are on his side, even when the chips are down. He must know that mistakes or problems will not be met with punishments but that they can be talked or worked through. The child also needs to understand that you know when he is doing well and that you will give him recognition for it. For years, Jack did not make any effort to take the lead in getting himself ready and settled for bed at night. Maybe this isn't such a big thing when you are in elementary school, but headed for middle school, he should start taking on more responsibility and develop a sense of self-modulation – when to get up, how to get ready for school on his own, making good choices for meals, and determining a reasonable bedtime and method for getting himself ready to sleep for the night.

I tried everything – charts, reward systems, point programs, and more. And I read every book on bedtime issues. But they all made one big assumption that wasn't true in my household – that the child was a willing participant in the bedtime routine. Jack's medication interferes with his sleep, and perhaps his own body chemistry does, too. Whatever the case, Jack is not tired at any reasonable bedtime hour, and no matter what I tried, I could not convince him that getting ten hours of sleep would ultimately serve him well.

I have an early-bird biological clock myself and can't wait to get to bed once 9 p.m. rolls around. I tried modeling this behavior for years for Jack. He wasn't biting. Then, weeks before he was to begin middle school, I saw something change. Jack began to think about bedtime differently. He began to think about what he had to do the following day. If there was somewhere he had to be in the morning, he realized that getting to bed earlier was a good idea.

Now, this wasn't anything different than what I had been saying all along. The only difference was that Jack had spent a summer in camp experiences, particularly Kanakuk, where the bedtime routine was modeled for him by cool college guys and peers. He could see how regular boys handled themselves at bedtime. He saw what happened to his cabin when he was late getting up and made everyone late for breakfast. That meant kitchen duty for the whole cabin. Not a good thing. Not a way to win cabin friends.

This was the event that changed Jack's bedtime routine. He gained a practical competency through the support and work of the camp counselors. They gave him the goal of getting up on time (clear expectations), reminded him what would happen in the morning to the cabin group if he wasn't up on time (anticipated the problem), and encouraged him to try and change his habits. Interestingly, Jack didn't have to get to sleep that much earlier to be able to get up on time. Getting to bed thirty minutes earlier was all he needed to be ready when the bugle blew. And when he stayed awake a little longer than the other boys? One of the counselors would stay up with him and read him the Bible. He came back from camp no longer asking me to make him a midnight snack but to read the Bible to him, thereby working on yet another piece of our vision for him.

LET YOUR CHILD KNOW HOW HE'S DOING

This past summer we spent a week in Sea Island, Georgia, where my husband and I have been vacationing since before our children were born. When we are there, Jack spends most of the day, every day, at the marina, fishing and crabbing off the dock. When he was young, this was a problem for our family. The marina is off by itself, and it is an extremely hot spot in an already hot place. No shade, hard wooden benches, and nothing but crab pots and fishing lines. John and I would trade off hour after hour of watching Jack at the dock and teaching him how to throw lines. Countless fishermen over the years have helped Jack retrieve a net, caught in the barnacles that are everywhere. It is more than a little thrilling that Jack is now old enough to spend the day as he wishes at Sea Island. He can join in any number of activities that are available for pre-teens, or he can hang out at the dock.

"I'm going to get a job at the dock this year," Jack announced as we were en route from his basketball camp to our family vacation.

"How are you so sure they are going to hire you?" I asked.

"Well, they've known me for years. And someone always needs a hand throwing a net out," he explained. I was amazed at how confident he sounded.

In between connecting flights I made a trip to the ladies room and promptly pulled out my cell phone. Soon I was talking to Marty at the marina, who, sure enough, remembered Jack.

"Marty, I am sure you can't hire an eleven-year-old, but Jack would love to work for you and I'd love for him to have the experience. How about if I pay you to pay him to work?"

Marty chuckled. "We would love to have him! I'm sorry we can't hire people under the age of sixteen, but we can certainly put him to work. Send him over at 9 a.m. after you get here."

I let Jack know that I had called the marina to see if they needed help and that they were looking for people. We went over some basic interview skills, and I added a few of my work philosophies:

"Give your boss more than she's expecting."

"Do the job to the best of your ability."

"Don't leave until the job is done."

Jack's first work experience was a win-win-win. The marina staff said he was terrific and bagged shrimp twice as fast as their regular employee. Jack was happy to be helping and earning money. And John and I were thrilled that he was getting his first taste of work in such a supportive and positive environment.

"That's terrific, Jack. You are doing a fine job" – Marty's praise knew no end. And if Jack needed a tweak or a slight tuning here or there, it was given gently and with lots of support.

STAY FIXED ON THE POTENTIAL

The Life Map unfolds as experience builds upon experience. There is a saying: "At birth our divine potential is folded up in us like a tent. It is life's purpose to unfold that tent."[26]

That potential can be coaxed into unfolding either like Charlie Brown or L.L. Bean. Remember how Charlie Brown used to wrestle with the kite that had a mind of its own? He inevitably ended up hanging upside-down from a tree with the kite having gotten the better of him. Only imagine if he tried to put a tent up. There would be arms and legs flying in every direction, unseen only because

---

[26] By Abbess Hildegard von Bingen, from *A Motivational Journey*, compiled by Jim Forrest (Grand Kaven, MI: Jim Forrest Seminars, n.d.), p. 115.

the tent would be covering him and flying in as many directions. In the end, both would be a tangled mess.

On the other hand, life's potential could unfold as cleanly as an L.L. Bean tent. A few years ago, a college friend invited me to join her and ten of her friends on a rafting trip down the Colorado River in the Grand Canyon. The first night, our guides explained the camping-out rules.

1. Everyone is responsible for their own equipment.

2. Everyone makes their own tent.

3. Everyone carries their own bag.

Wait. Back to rule number two. I have this fear of pitching a tent. It looks hard. Very hard. Almost impossible. My friend Valerie and I looked at each other and then up at the sky. It was clear.

"It is *not* going to rain," I declared.

"No way," she confirmed.

"No need for the tent," I determined.

"Absolutely not," she agreed.

We unrolled our sleeping bags and settled down for the night, drifting off to sleep under a million stars.

"Anne, wake up." Someone was shaking me. As I started to wake, I felt something cold dropping on my face. "It's starting to rain," Val said.

Oh, great. No tent. We ran up from where we had situated ourselves to wake up Sheila, the gal in our group who knew how to pitch a tent.

"Sheila, can you help us? We need to pitch our tent and quick!" Val begged. Good-naturedly, Sheila rolled out of her sleep sack and got up to demonstrate. Valerie and I were all ears. We knew we couldn't pull this stunt again. Funny enough, it was not so hard, once Sheila broke the process down for us. Five steps. Once I got over my preconception that pitching a tent took a Ph.D. and applied myself to learning its mystery, it was no harder than assembling a kid's toy.

The Life Map takes the mystery out of figuring out the best way to help your child achieve his potential. By developing a vision and formulating plans that support that vision, your child's potential can unfold as easily as that L.L. Bean tent.

Now that you have a better understanding of what the Life Map is about, let's take a look at how it operates in real life. As you see how the plan works in everyday life, try to imagine an overlay of the deep understanding of your child that we explored in Section 1, the self-reflection that we talked about in Section 2, and the commitment to doing your part to make the team as effective as possible that we reviewed in Section 3. The better you are at these things, the more process-driven the plan will become.

THE BOTTOM LINE

- When you formulate the plans, or missions, to help your child reach the vision for him, think in terms of what can be accomplished in immediate, medium-term, and longer-term timeframes.

- Your role is to teach, support, encourage, and coach your child so that his full potential can be brought out.

- Crafting a program that will lead your child to reach his potential should be no more difficult than unfolding that L.L. Bean tent.

- The power of the Life Map approach lies in its ability to keep you focused on what is *inside* the tent. While everyone else is asking you what is wrong with the tent and wondering how you can get it fixed so that it looks and operates like every other tent, the Life Map remains fixed on the vision.

SECTION 2

PUTTING THE PLAN INTO PRACTICE

CHAPTER 1

HOW THE PLAN WORKS

Developing the Life Map in Eight Easy Steps

CHAPTER 2

MAKING IT WORK

Partners Until the End

CHAPTER 3

LIFE MAPPING LESSONS

A Few Words of Wisdom

CHAPTER 1

How the Plan Works

Developing the Life Map in Eight Easy Steps

The Life Map is not something you decide to work on a rainy afternoon when there is nothing better to do. It is not something you create and then put away never to look at again. The Life Map should be well thought out and include the input of those who work closely with your child, including your child, and it should encompass all aspects of your child's life. It is something that grows out of observation, conversation, and careful thinking. And now, how to go about developing a Life Map.

Step 1: Articulate the Vision

If you have never done any vision setting for yourself, your family, or your children, now is the time to start. If you have a spouse, significant other or someone who is closely involved with your child, agree on a time when you have a few uninterrupted hours or agree to do it over a period of a few weekends or days. Put the time aside on the calendar and treat it as you would a real work meeting, choosing a quiet place with no interruptions. Perhaps your library has a meeting room that you can reserve or a quiet corner where you won't disturb anyone or be disturbed.

As you go through the process of thinking through what is most important to your family, you may want to get some outside input. Talking about this with trusted friends, family members, and those you respect can give you new perspectives and ideas. This is not about painting a specific picture of one sort or another. At the end of your exercise, don't expect to have a vision of a particular house, with a car and a dog and some children running around outside. The children shouldn't be wearing nametags indicating what college they will go to and what field they will pursue as adults. Try for a vision such as "To be happy." This is on a whole different dimension than "To live in a 3,000-square-foot house."

Once you have a vision, developing the guts of the Life Map can begin. The rest of the plan beyond the vision should be revisited annually. It may be easiest to follow the academic calendar, since you will be gathering some of the same data that will be used for your child's IEP.

STEP 2: GATHER INFORMATION AND SYNTHESIZE INPUT

Three men were blindfolded and each led to a different part of an elephant. "This is a tree!" said the first, feeling the animal's stiff, upright trunk. "It must be a baby calf," said the next, rubbing his hand against the soft underbelly of the gentle giant. "I know it is a hippopotamus!" the third said with great certainty, feeling the roughest part of the hind leg.

In the above example, notice how different each person's conclusion was, based upon his specific experience. Similarly, we may miss some valuable opportunities if we look at our child from only our own perspective. Right from the start, gather information from those who know your child and whose opinions you respect. (Appendix B provides a simple questionnaire that you can ask each person to fill out that will provide you with information to help you formulate some missions, goals, strategies, and tactics.)

Don't be rigid about how you gather the information. Some people may prefer the questionnaire so that they can fill it out on their own time. Others may want to share some thoughts over a Coke. Do whatever works best. Think broadly about who might have good information to contribute. One of the most valuable members of Jack's team is Julien, the now sixteen-year-old mentor who has taught Jack how to be "a regular boy" (by Jack's account) by just being his friend. Julien has his own ongoing agenda for what Jack needs to be working on and learning and makes no bones about making sure he learns it – from how to treat girls to fishing for bass.

Ask those whom you are requesting information from (which should include your school-based team members) to think about the past year and to articulate your child's gains and accomplishments, his strengths, and issues that were resolved as well as those that remain unresolved, and to relate any strategies and tactics that were particularly successful for them. Share with them that you are developing the Life Map and invite them to propose preliminary goals for the coming year.

Finally, and very important, talk to your child about his passions and interests and what he wants from life. The older the child and the more emotionally mature he is, the more active he can be in this process.

Once you've gathered this information, take a piece of paper and at the top write down the major categories of your child's life. Then record the input under the respective headings. You are looking for major themes and a consensus of opinions in the areas of overall development – social, behavioral/emotional, academic, physical, and outside interests. Identify the major areas that seem to be shared. Once you have written down everyone's input, including your own, walk away for a few days. Let it rest and settle in. It is good to get some distance and perspective rather than rushing through this exercise.

Step 3: Develop the Mission(s)

Once you return to the information, get ready to develop one or two missions. The mission is the stairway of accomplishments that will get you to the vision. Missions are the overarching categories that are needed to accomplish the vision. You should probably have a mission for each of the major areas of your child's life: social, emotional, and academic.

Step 4: Map out the Goals, Strategies, and Tactics

Flowing right out of the missions will be the goals, strategies, and tactics that will help achieve the missions. The goals are more specific and immediate. Every goal should be one that the child can reasonably achieve within one year, provided he is supported by the right strategies and tactics.

It is tempting to become overenthusiastic about goals. Resist the urge to go after more than four goals a year. It is far better to focus on a few goals than to use a shotgun approach and only gain a little ground in a lot of different areas. This shouldn't stop you from writing down as many goals as you can think of, however. But then go back and be tough – prioritize. Ask, what are the goals that, if met, would make the biggest difference in your child's life and open a whole other set of opportunities to him?

As you identify each goal and think about possible strategies and tactics, think also about every place in your child's life where goals can be worked on. Think comprehensively. Take a look at all the possible places that your child could be working on reaching his goals, sometimes without even knowing it!

Oh, Oh! The Places the Goals Will Go!

Your child's goals can be worked on in all of the following places:

Home	Playground
School	Mealtimes
Sports team	Social events
Extracurricular lessons	The community
Religious education	Doctor's visits

STEP 5: GAIN CONSENSUS AROUND THE PROPOSED PLAN

Sure, you've developed the plan for your child, but you want the team to be comfortable with it, too. It is probably easiest to send out a short letter to those you want to buy into the plan, showing them the preliminary goals that you are thinking of along with possible strategies and tactics that they have suggested or that you have thought of. Invite them to write in strategies and tactics that they think they could employ when working with the child.

Step 6: Establish a Process for Carrying out the Plan

You don't want to make carrying out the plan seem like such a big deal to people that they start shaking their heads, saying, "Oh, no. We are already implementing a plan," or "That's not my job to implement a plan." The plan is in your head and hands, and you must convey it in a practical, no-fuss manner. You want to make three main points:

1. "Here are the goals that we will be working on with Jack in the coming months. We appreciate your input in helping us establish some priority around all of his needs. If you can keep these in mind as you work with him that would be terrific."

2. "If you see Jack slipping in general or not making progress toward any of these goals, please let us know."

3. "If you need help from us or if we can do anything to make your job easier, please let us know. We're here to support you."

Step 7: Implement the Plan

The Life Map gets implemented exactly as its name implies – twenty-four hours a day, seven days a week. I think about life in terms of these chunks of time:

• School

• Connective Time – Meals, baths, getting ready to go places, going places, getting ready for bed

• Advancing the Plan – All the time that the child is awake and not in school or busy with daily life (connective time activities). This is his "down time" or free time and the time that you need to think long and hard about. What is better – letting him hang out playing on the computer, going for an extra therapy, session, or playing a board game with him where you are "secretly" working on the goals? Resist the urge to let him go with the flow of the day and be deliberate about the activities he is engaged in and what, from your Life Map perspective, is their purpose.

• Sleep

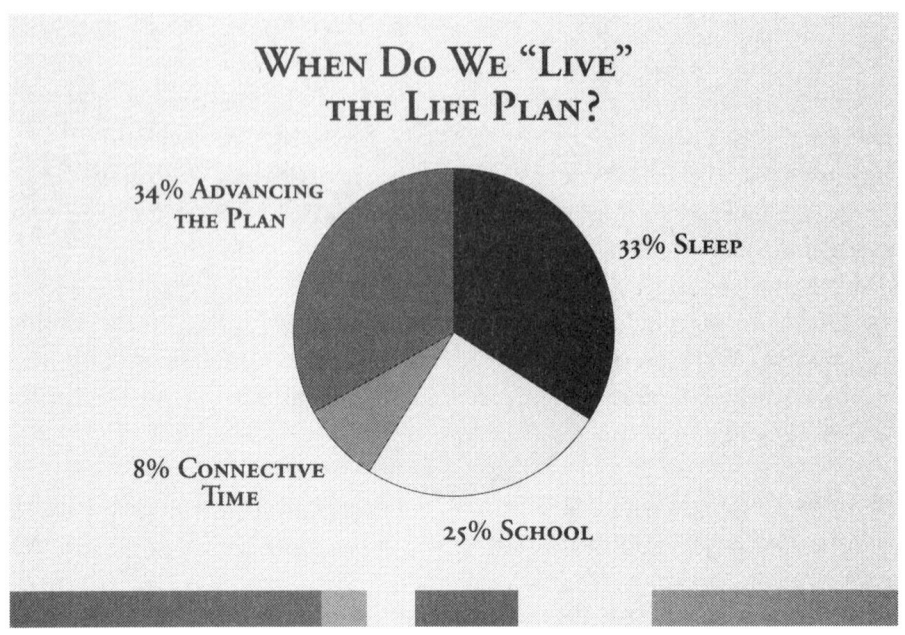

WHEN DO WE "LIVE" THE LIFE PLAN?

34% ADVANCING THE PLAN

33% SLEEP

8% CONNECTIVE TIME

25% SCHOOL

This might sound exhausting, and, at first, it does require a bit of an adjustment in your thinking. There is an opportunity in virtually every moment of your child's day, except when he is sleeping. But, if you think about it, even sleeping is a part of the plan. Anyone who questions the importance of a good night's sleep for mood and coping ability need only observe an overtired child.

Here is where you want to think about balance. Take a look at the major goals you have established. Is there an opportunity to work on them in every setting of the day? For an example, take a goal that we want our children to master as they become older and that they have moved beyond the basics on: initial greetings. As we get older, initial greetings are where we are quickly judged. "First impressions are lasting ones" is not an idle phrase; it is true that a first impression can often get you in the door or close it abruptly. Unfortunately, greetings can be among the biggest challenges for some kids, such as the ones who struggle with eye contact.

I am sure Jack has long ago tuned me out when it comes to initial greetings. "Say hello and look him in the eye, Jack" has probably gone in one ear and out the other a million times in his life time. But working on this skill takes on a new level when it's coming at Jack from all sides and in different ways. Julien, in his teenage way, can say, "Come on, Jack, say hello and talk to me instead of telling me what you want to do when I walk in the door!" and make the point that we don't start out with a demand the minute we see someone. The speech therapist at school can spend the first twenty minutes of a session walking around with Jack practicing how many people he can greet and have two minutes of small talk with, making it a game. The basketball coach and Sunday School teacher can make sure that they get a decent hello and deliberately ask Jack how his weekend is going before he joins the class, again reinforcing what we are working on. It can happen easily just by you asking each person your child sees on a regular basis if he or she would help you by doing x, y, z as you are working on a particular goal.

Life Mapping takes a look at every aspect of your child's day and asks the question, "Are the activities that he is doing supporting and building toward the goals and vision that we have set for our child?" The answer should be a resounding "Yes!" If your child's goal for the next six months is working on "learning to share with others," you had better have in place activities that give him the opportunity to practice this competency – with the necessary supports – at home, in his outside therapies, and in his extracurricular activities. Life Mapping makes sure that you are being intentional about how your child spends his time and that it is being spent on getting him to the place that is best for him to some day be.

STEP 8: CHART PROGRESS

Charting the progress of the plan should be no different from a process standpoint than how a good IEP is carried out during the year. You will have three or four goals written down with the key strategies and tactics laid out by setting. Every month, pull this sheet out and check in with the folks who are working with your child in each of the areas. Ask them how your child is doing against the goals and think about your own observations. Make adjustments if progress isn't evident. Your child's rate of progress will be uneven and will probably include some backward movement; this is to be expected. But over time, you should see a gradual move forward. If not, go back to the drawing board.

Remember our discussion a few sections back about process? Well, carrying out the Life Map is a process. Once you go from plan to process, you may find that things do not go as perfectly as you had hoped. That is to be expected and should not throw you.

- Take time to develop the Life Map with your child. The first step is to develop a vision that is appropriate and attainable for your child. Also talk over the vision with your spouse and others whom you trust and who can give you new perspectives and ideas.

- Gather information from those who work closely with your child to develop the missions that will support the vision. These should be accomplishments you think the child can achieve in three to five years. The goals, strategies, and tactics will flow from the missions and should be attainable within a year. Revisit all these steps except the vision annually to see if any adjustments are necessary.

- The Life Map should be implemented twenty-four hours a day, seven days a week, in every aspect of the child's life.

CHAPTER 2

MAKING IT WORK
Partners Until the End

It is time to cycle back to where it all began – with the child. You can have the best Life Map possible, be blessed with an awesome team, and be the most on-top-of-it parent imaginable, but if your child isn't a partner in the program, carrying out the Life Map will be very, very slow going. Depending upon your child's functioning level and age, his degree of cooperation may be low. Don't despair. During these times, the Life Map is more important than ever because it will allow you to stay very, very focused.

Even if your child has good cognitive functioning and cooperation levels, don't think that you can merely walk up to him and say, "Hey, let's review this Life Map that we created for you. Want to see how you can do your part in it?" If you do this, you can be sure that your child will *not* be working on anything you wanted him to work on, particularly if he is in or near the teenage years.

So, how are we going to get our children to be partners?

Offer Encouragement

It's as simple as letting your child know that you are on his side, that you notice when he does a good job, and that what he does matters to you. When you encourage your child, be specific with your praise so that he knows exactly what behavior it was that made you proud.

Reward Good Decisions, Behaviors, and Actions

Support your encouragement with ample words and actions that let your child know that what he did was terrific. Make both nonverbal and verbal expressions of support part of your regular interaction with your child. This may seem obvious, but I find that I sometimes have to remind myself to make sure Jack knows that I have noticed what he has accomplished. Depending upon the child and the behavior system you use (if there is one), you may want to give your child a concrete reward. Unless your child is on a specific reward system, this does not have to be on any regular schedule. Once in a while, if Jack does something unexpected and other-oriented, I stop everything and take him out for an ice cream cone or to the movies to really let him know how special what he did was.

You do not want to send a message that doing good deeds or behaving correctly means that the child will be "paid off" for it; that is the danger of linking a concrete or tangible reward too often. However, if you keep the reward to something that is mainly another opportunity for developing a positive connection with him and something that he will find enjoyable, you will set in his mind, hopefully, the importance of what he did. When you take him out for that ice cream cone, you might say to him something like, "I just want you to know how much I appreciated and liked what you did today and wanted to spend special time with you because I am so proud of you."

Shift Your Mind-Set

If your mind is in a negative place – if things are not going so well today, this week, or this month – it's up to you to get it back on track. If you expect your child to respect and trust you – which is what partnering is all about – he must be able to see you as consistent, dependable, and truthful. If you exude an attitude that says, "Hey, I believe in you no matter what is going on at this time," he gains the confidence that you are here for the long haul.

Build in Success

No one wants to be in a relationship where he feels that he can't carry his own weight or that he is not a valued partner. Build in experiences and opportunities for the child to be successful, to help build his self-confidence and his confidence in his relationship with you.

Offer Unconditional Listening, Unconditional Love

Joe White, the president of Kanakuk-Kanakomo Kamps, is no stranger to listening, with over 14,000 campers in attendance each summer. Joe believes that listening is a central ingredient in any dialogue with a child.[27] When a child has a problem, he tells the child that he would like to ask him three questions and that he would like the child to think of three different solutions to his problem. What Joe is trying to do is to help the child work toward discovering his own solution to the problem. Obviously, this is a technique that is best suited for higher-functioning children and children nearing middle school age.

The three questions are:

1. What is wrong?

2. What are you feeling?

3. What are you going to do about it?

Joe has three ground rules that must be in place for the communication method to work effectively. First, you must be empathetic. You must show this empathy not just with your words but with your eyes, your body language, and your expressions. The child must feel that you truly and really understand him and are empathetic to what he is feeling.

Second, you must not offer any premature advice or jump to conclusions before you have asked the three questions. What the child answers the first time may not be the real answer to the question. Take the time to listen fully and reflect upon all three answers before you offer your thoughts.

---

[27] Joe White, *What Kids Wish Parents Knew About Parenting* (West Monroe, LA: Howard Publishing Co., 1998), pp. 59-61.

Third, do not say anything judgmental or negative. Statements such as "How could you do that?" or "Why did you say that?" will put the child on the defensive and close the communication door immediately.

Learning to ask questions and to listen will open the way to dialoguing. And what better way to build a partnership than through strong communication? If you haven't figured it out yet, learning to be a good listener and showering your child with love is all about heart-set, and making sure it is in the right place.

WHERE DOES YOUR PARTNERSHIP STAND?

Take a look at the following statements and see if you can determine where the strengths and weaknesses in your partnership with your child lie.

HOW IS YOUR RELATIONSHIP WITH YOUR CHILD?

How do you think your child would respond to the following statements? Read each statement and then respond by circling a number. 5 = strongly agree and 1 = strongly disagree.

1. My mother knows me very well.
   5   4   3   2   1
2. My father knows me very well.
   5   4   3   2   1
3. If I have a problem, I feel that I can go to at least one of my parents.
   5   4   3   2   1
4. When I talk with my parents, I feel they listen to me.
   5   4   3   2   1
5. My relationship with my mom is very good.
   5   4   3   2   1
6. My relationship with my dad is very good.
   5   4   3   2   1

Add up your scores. The higher the score, the greater the likelihood that you are partnering with your child. It might be interesting to give these six statements to your child and see how his responses compare with how you think you are doing.

Who Said It Would Be Easy?

Much of what goes on with your relationship with your child is out of your control. His attitudes, feelings, and sense of his relationship with you is largely a product of his own mind-set and heart-set. As tough as it can sometimes be, you are the adult and the one who needs to continually model what a healthy relationship should be. Even if it doesn't seem to be making a dent today, you are planting the seeds that will eventually take root and influence his development.

THE BOTTOM LINE

- Your child is part of the team and a very important partner in the process.

- A strong relationship with your child doesn't just happen. Your support, encouragement, and unconditional love, shown through your actions and your words, build the partnership.

- No matter what your child's functioning level is, a relationship is possible.

CHAPTER 3

LIFE MAPPING LESSONS
A Few Words of Wisdom

Cracking the mystery of how your child sees the world does not happen overnight. And it is not a task for someone who doesn't have the words *persistence* and *patience* in their vocabulary. The first thing to figure out is how removed your child is from the rest of the world. Another way to think about this is to ask yourself, "How does my child view the world and see himself in connection to it?"

PLANTING SEEDS EARLY

If you have a child who is in a totally self-absorbed stage, don't even think about teaching him about the social world. The first step is to make him aware of himself. This has to start with the tiniest demand of him and then sticking with the behavior that you want. For example, at the age of ten months, Jack was able to hurl himself out of his crib and escape to freedom. For a child who never slept, this was not a good thing. He would crawl to our bedroom and wake me up by sitting on my face, poking my arm, and doing whatever it took to wake me up. The waking-up thing was still happening at age ten.

Totally exhausted we acknowledged that we had to get some of this sleep issue under control, and I was propelled into action. Our child had to realize that just because he was awake didn't mean I had to be awake. I would lie there, morning after morning, while he tried to get me to wake up and pretend to continue to sleep. I had a timer next to the bed and would tell Jack that I was going to sleep for five more minutes and that he had to wait for the timer to ring. I tried this for weeks. Jack continued to poke and prod. During the day, when things were calm, I would bring up the situation and tell Jack that I understood he wasn't tired but that I needed my sleep. He gave no response, and I had no idea if my conversation made any dent – until one day he came in to our bedroom, took one look at me sleeping, and went back to his room to play.

This story holds a large lesson that I have found over and over, particularly as Jack gets older. It is *critical* to have a conversation about what the right thing to do is and what your expectations are for your child. You may think he is not hearing a single word or understanding you a bit. But you are planting seeds. It may not seem as if anything is happening underneath the surface, but you might be surprised. The seeds you plant will eventually be harvested.

In this example of waking me up every morning, I don't think that Jack's behavior changed because he learned what it means to be a considerate person. What I did at this stage was merely train him and expose him to the language and concept of consideration for others – not knowing if any of it made a dent. I had to continue reinforcing the importance of not waking me up. It wasn't until this past year, now that Jack is eleven, that on most days he didn't wake me and for the right reasons. His world has changed enough so that he understands and respects that my needs are different from his. Yet, even as I write this, I am chuckling because yesterday morning, Martin Luther King Day, a day when I was looking forward to everyone in the house, including me, sleeping in, I was woken by a hearty "Top of the morning to you!" by Jack at 7:00 a.m. At least he went down and made his own breakfast when I asked him to let me sleep.

Planting seeds is just one part of the equation though. You might think of it as your offensive plan. The other side is that you must be able to see the world as your child sees it. This will help you enormously in several ways. First, you will know what issues you have to work on. For me, after examining the "why" in why Jack was waking me up and realizing he had no concept of my needs being different from his and no sense of consideration, I could begin to work on those elements. I could come up with a plan to work toward the behavior that would be acceptable, and I could plant seeds of information about the right thing to do. And at some point, I told Jack what he had to begin to do to empower him to overcome it, as best he could.

Never Say "Never"

Jack has always had a significant problem getting to sleep. In the early years, he wouldn't fall asleep until 1 a.m. and was up again at 4. His psychiatrist has tried different medications – mild sleep inducers and even Benadryl – but after a while, the drugs lose their ability to help Jack get to sleep. When Jack was in fourth grade, I decided that it was time to go after a few of these life behaviors that Jack would have to get a handle on as he grew older. I already pictured him as one of those quirky science professors, the one in the lab with the lone light burning at ungodly hours. I felt that I just had to get him to develop some fundamental life habits, the first being getting to bed at a reasonable hour.

The *only* thing that helped Jack get to sleep was me lying next to him. I knew that wasn't a good habit to develop. I asked Jack why it was that he was able to get to sleep when I was lying next to him. Without hesitation, Jack said "body heat." "I'm cold and need your body heat to get to sleep." That was the most unexpected answer I could imagine, since the boy had two down comforters on his bed. I thought about that for a moment and decided there might be a sensory issue underneath it all. Maybe an electric blanket would fit the bill.

The next day I raced out to get the blanket. Wouldn't it be amazing if a $99 investment did the trick? Believe it or not, it seems to. Although Jack still gets to sleep later than I'd like (somewhere between 10 and 11:30 p.m.), at least it's on the right side of midnight. Who would've guessed?

The blanket did the trick – for a while that is. It would have been too easy to say that this solved the problem forever. It helped for a time until something else threw Jack's system out of whack. The lesson here is to keep looking for answers, and when one thing doesn't work, try something different.

WHEN ALL IS SAID AND DONE

The reality of life with children is that there is no bottom line. There never is. There is a line that is constantly changing. And for your one-of-a-kind child sometimes it's hard to figure out where the line is. To truly unfold your child's tent, you need to understand him, work hard to make the plan work, never give up on him – and most of all – love him for who he is.

THE BOTTOM LINE

- The world can't slow to your child's pace. The more tools that you can give your child, the more he will be able to adapt to situations and become empowered.

- The more that you prepare the environment, work with the team, and provide your child with skills and competencies, the more he will be able to manage his world independently. However, this does not promise success in all situations. New situations will trip him up. Be prepared, knowing that this is just part of the journey.

- If a disaster strikes, don't despair or give up. Keep your perspective, remember this is just one moment in time, and try a new approach.

Nothing is hard to those whose will is set on it,
especially if it be a thing to be done out of love ...
If you want to bring anything to a successful conclusion,
you must accommodate yourself to the task, not the task to yourself.

– St. Ignatius Loyola

BIBLIOGRAPHY

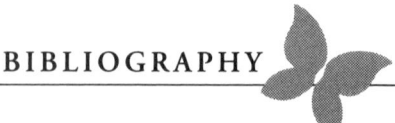

Addison, A. (2003). *One Small Starfish.* Arlington, TX: Future Horizons.

Brooks, R., & Goldstein, S. (2001). *Raising Resilient Children.* New York: McGraw-Hill.

Covey, S. (1989). *Seven Habits of Highly Effective People.* New York: Fireside Books.

Dobson, J. (2001). *Bringing up Boys: Practical Advice and Encouragement for Those Shaping the Next Generation of Men.* Carol Stream, IL: Tyndale House Publishing.

Family Educational Rights Privacy Law. www.ed.gov/policy/gen/guid/fpco/ferpa

Forrest, J. (n.d.). *A Motivational Journey.* Grand Kaven, MI: Jim Forrest Seminars.

Gravelle, K. et al. (1998). *What's Going on Down There? Answers to Questions Boys Find Difficult to Ask.* New York: Walker Publishing Company.

IDEA www.ed.gov/policy/speced/guid/idea/idea2004/html.

Kencel, R., & Eberhardt, S. (in press). *I Only Have a Minute So This Better Be Good.* Greenwich, CT.

Leman, K. (1998). *The New Birth Order Book.* Grand Rapids, MI: Baker Book House Co.

Manning, W. D. (2003, November). Adolescent Well-Being in Cohabiting, Married and Single-Parent Families. *American Journal of Marriage and Family, 65*(4).

Maxwell, J.C. (2002). *17 Essential Qualities of a Team Player: Becoming the Kind of Person Every Team Wants.* Nashville, TN: Thomas Nelson Publishers.

Palladino, L. J. (1997). *The Edison Trait.* New York: Times Books.

Reitz, A. L. (n.d.). *A Strengths-Based Approach to Treatment.* Quincy, MA: Child Welfare League of America.

Wallace, M. (1989). *Birth Order Blues.* New York: Henry Holt and Co.

White, J. (1998). *What Kids Wish Parents Knew About Parenting.* West Monroe, LA: Howard Publishing Co.

QUARTERLY MEMO – SAMPLE

Anne Addison
(Your address goes here)

August 28, 2002

Dear Mrs. Connors and other teachers working with Jack,

This is an "Introduction to Jack" letter that I prepare each year to give teachers a quick look at Jack's special needs and characteristics. The strides he has made since coming to North Street just a year and a half ago have been incredible, and we trust and know that this year will be the same. So, first and foremost, thank you for all your efforts on Jack's behalf.

Quick Overview of Jack's Needs

Jack has ADHD and features of Asperger Syndrome. He doesn't have the narrow focus and obsessiveness that are two of the hallmarks of Asperger Syndrome which is a social disability in that people do not pick up social cues, have poor pragmatic skills (tending to focus on their own interests), have poor eye contact and poor social common sense.

For Jack, we are always reminding him to make and keep eye contact, and we work on social appropriateness primarily by putting people (including older boys) in his path who model correct behavior. Marty Clarke was a huge influence on Jack last year and may play that role again this year. The two boys will be taking tennis lessons together weekly, so we hope the friendship will continue to grow.

If I had to select four highest priority social-oriented goals, I would say:

1. Eye contact

2. Listening and accepting the other person's perspective

3. Cooperation with adults and peers in terms of being flexible, working well in a team, etc.

4. Flexibility – being able to move on when the task is not completed fully or not completed to the level of perfection that Jack finds acceptable (Mrs. Karfopoulos can give you more information on this).

In terms of academic goals, Jack needs significant help with expository writing from the development of ideas to drawing conclusions. This is a huge goal for us in fifth grade.

In terms of his ADHD, impulsivity and hyperactivity are the two areas that Jack struggles with the most. He saw the doctor who manages his medication, Concerta, today and she decided to increase the dose slightly. We are depending on you to tell us if Jack is sustaining focus during the day and is attentive. If he appears subdued, dopey, or lethargic, please let us know immediately – though I know it's tough since you don't have a "before" benchmark.

Summer

Jack spent seven weeks at a sleep-away camp in the Adirondack Mountains. I am including the camp rating form for you to see how Jack performed. Overall, they said he had improved significantly vs. the previous summer but needs to work on the social and cooperative skills that I mentioned above.

OUR PHILOSOPHY

I believe that as parents we have two jobs as members of the team supporting Jack: (1) work on the goals given in the IEP at home and provide outside experiences where these goals can be worked on, and (2) be a coordinator/communication liaison for the team. Please know that we are the kind of parents that believe in working as partners with you and catching things early, as in, almost immediately. If at any time, you see anything that is concerning, let us know via e-mail, voice mail, or phone call so that we can begin to address it with you.

I would like for you to forward me your e-mail addresses so if things come up, I can easily contact you.

As Jack has gotten "healthier," he has discovered so many interests. This year he is on a fall travel soccer team, will take tennis and squash lessons, is in the church choir, and is taking violin lessons. He also hopes to be in the school orchestra. Whether Jack can sustain this level of outside activity remains to be seen. He did so last year but the homework load was very manageable. These experiences give him a chance to work on social skills and I work carefully with the coaches and instructors so that they know exactly what the issues are.

However, if you see that Jack is not getting work completed or is overtired, please let me know so that I can adjust what we are doing.

HOT SPOTS

Here are a few things to be aware of:

1. Jack has a huge sleeping problem – difficulty falling to sleep. He was often late to school last year since he sometimes can't get to sleep until 2 a.m. We are trying not to use prescription medication to solve this as it can become addictive. So far since July, he has been sleeping better and he knows getting to school on time is important – if you can make his timely arrival noticed and a big deal, it will reinforce the fact that this is a big priority (it's even in the IEP as a goal!).

2. Being calm and patient is much more effective than being rattled and impatient with Jack – he is very sensitive and falls apart if he feels pressure. If he interrupts too often or does something irksome, perhaps you can have a special hand signal or something similar.

3. Overall, Jack is very sensitive and very concerned that he has a good reputation and is seen as a nice kid.

4. Jack loves to learn but can become overwhelmed if the environment is too loud or busy.

I could go on and on, but this is, I'm sure, quite enough.

Thank you and feel free to contact me. I would appreciate it if you could write me a short e-mail or have Jill Flood do so every few days so I know how everything is going and if I need to talk/reinforce anything at home.

Many thanks!

Anne Addison

P.S. The homework for summer is in the backpack.

APPENDIX B

Life Mapping Form

Respondent's Name _____

Date _____

1. What are the key strengths of this child?

_____

_____

_____

2. What are your key areas of concern for this child?

_____

_____

_____

3. What special passions, interests, talents do you see in this child?

_____

_____

_____

4. What do you see as the biggest emotional challenges affecting this child?

_____

_____

_____

5. What do you see as the biggest social challenges affecting this child?

_____

_____

_____

6. Where has this child made the greatest gains with you this year?

_____

_____

_____

7. What do you think were the major factors contributing to that gain?

_____

_____

_____

8. What kind of person (qualities, attributes, personality traits) do you think works most successfully with this child and what kind of person does this child learn the most from?

_____

_____

_____

9. Is there anything that you would like to add?

_____

_____

_____

Thank you for helping us with this information.

Share Your Stories

Do you have stories of empowerment and achieving potential when you thought it couldn't be done? I would love to hear them and consider using them in my next book. Please feel free to write to me at <u>www.anneaddison.com</u>.

INDEX

Life Map Offers Parents an Important Tool for Helping Their Child Prosper and Grow

Unfolding the Tent: Advocating for Your One-Of-A-Kind Child is for parents of children with behavioral, attentional, developmental and learning needs. Because these children do not follow a typical developmental path, it is unrealistic to think that they can grow to become the best that they can be without careful attention to their unique needs and gifts. Using strategic planning methodology, Anne Addison introduces the Life Map, which draws upon the child's strengths and passions and takes into consideration the unique way in which he sees the world. Parents learn methods to become effective coaches, case managers and members of the team supporting their child. In addition, exercises throughout the book encourage parents to examine their parenting style and their role in their child's life. Filled with personal stories and case studies to highlight key points, this book takes a proactive and positive approach to helping children "be the best they can be."

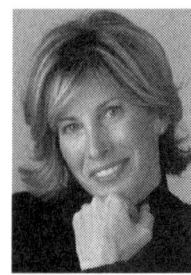

About the Author

Anne Addison is the author of *One Small Starfish: A Mother's Everyday Advice, Survival Tactics & Wisdom for Raising a Special Needs Child.* She has lectured at conferences throughout the country and her writings are featured in numerous magazines. She runs a private company and is a member of education and health-care related boards. She lives in Connecticut with her husband and two children.